An Integrated Approach to Nutrition and Exercise

An Integrated Approach to Nutrition and Exercise

Edited by Fred Collins

STATES
ACADEMIC PRESS
www.statesacademicpress.com

Published by States Academic Press,
109 South 5th Street,
Brooklyn, NY 11249, USA
www.statesacademicpress.com

An Integrated Approach to Nutrition and Exercise
Edited by Fred Collins

International Standard Book Number: 978-1-63989-045-3 (Hardback)

Cataloging-in-Publication Data

An integrated approach to nutrition and exercise / edited by Fred Collins.
p. cm.
Includes bibliographical references and index.
ISBN 978-1-63989-045-3
1. Nutrition. 2. Physiology. 3. Diet. 4. Food habits. 5. Exercise.
6. Physical fitness. I. Collins, Fred.
QP141 .I58 2022
613.2--dc23

TABLE OF CONTENTS

PREFACE

The purpose of the book is to provide a glimpse into the dynamics and to present opinions and studies of some of the scientists engaged in the development of new ideas in the field from very different standpoints. This book will prove useful to students and researchers owing to its high content quality.

Nutrition is a fundamental biochemical and physiological process intrinsic to all living organisms. Essential nutrients present in food are vital for humans to support good health and life. In the absence of the right nutrition, humans become susceptible to diseases such as anemia, blindness, obesity, metabolic syndrome, and even preterm birth and stillbirth. Nutrition must be supported by regular and targeted exercise for fitness and overall health. These physical activities may be targeted to specific outcomes, such as muscle development, prevention of aging, weight loss, or slowing of aging. This book studies, analyses and upholds the pillars of nutrition and exercise and their utmost significance in modern times. Most of the topics introduced herein cover modern perspectives on diet, nutrition, and physical fitness. This book is a complete source of knowledge on the present status of these domains.

At the end, I would like to appreciate all the efforts made by the authors in completing their chapters professionally. I express my deepest gratitude to all of them for contributing to this book by sharing their valuable works. A special thanks to my family and friends for their constant support in this journey.

Editor

1

Dietary Intakes and Nutritional Status of a Greek Team of Female Volleyball Players

Galanis Nikiforos[1], Kleftouris George[2], Alafropatis Ilias[1], Oral Onur[3], Tsiridis Eleftherios[1], Sayegh Fares[1], and Kirkos John[1]

[1]Division of Sports Medicine, Department of Orthopaedics, Papageorgiou General Hospital, Medical School, Aristotle University of Thessaloniki, Greece
[2]Royal Lancaster Infirmary University Hospital, NHS trust, Lancaster, UK
[3] School of Physical Education and Sports, Ege University, Izmir, Turkey

Corresponding Author: Galanis Nikiforos; email: ngalanismed@gmail.com

Abstract

Aim: The purpose of this study was to assess the dietary intakes and nutritional status of a nationally ranked team of female volleyball players. **Methods:** The subjects completed a general history questionnaire and 7-day food and physical activity records. Anthropometric measurements included height, weight, triceps and subscapular skinfolds and mid-upper-arm circumference. Biochemical assessment included parameters for protein, lipid, and iron status. **Results:** All subjects had normal menstrual cycles and body fat values (27 %) at levels higher than for optimum performance. Most were in negative energy balance and had low energy (30 kcal/kg/d), carbohydrate (3.8 g/kg/d) and protein (1.0 g/kg/d) intakes. Fat intakes were high (39 %) and micronutrient intakes were below recommended levels, except for vitamin C, vitamin B12 and niacin. Biochemical indices were normal except for iron and lipid status of some players. **Conclusion:** These results indicate that the players of this team have dietary intakes that place them at risk for nutritional shortages and compromised performance; they need professional counseling regarding nutrition practices for optimum health and performance.

Keywords: exercise, nutrition, volleyball, anthropometry, biochemical assessment, macronutrients, micronutrients

1. Introduction

Volleyball is one of the most popular sports among females in Greece. It is one of the three main team sports included in the curriculum of Greek schools, besides soccer and basketball. Volleyball is an activity requiring combined physical and mental abilities such as explosive strength, agility, a high level of concentration and skill. As an activity, it relies mostly on the anaerobic energy system though aerobic endurance is important for recovery between points, stamina and tolerance to heat [25]. Training includes skill, strength and conditioning programs. In addition, having reduced body fat levels can help improve the athletes? speed and jumping ability. Volleyball players need powerful legs to assist with jumping and strong upper bodies to develop power for spiking, serving and blocking. Competitive female volleyball athletes face increased demands for energy and nutrients to support heavy training, along with a need to lower body fat to low-moderate levels for optimum performance [5].

Female athletes participating in sports that emphasize leanness (eg gymnastics, figure skating, and cross-country running) generally report energy and nutrient intakes below recommended levels and lower than those of non-athletic females. This is thought to be due to weight control practices common among these athletes while neuropsychopharmacological parameters and disorders are under investigation [1, 3, 31], (da Silva et al. 2015), and [30].

Dietary intakes and eating behaviors of female athletes participating in sports with less emphasis on low body weight (e.g. swimming, rowing, soccer, basketball and volleyball) are also reported to be sub-optimal [2, 11, 12, 18, 20, 31].

This might be due to lack of professional nutritional support of female athletes along with heavy training and improper body image perceptions [2, 28]. The main objectives of the present study were to examine the dietary intakes and nutritional status of a team of female Greek volleyball players and some of the risk factors related to their nutritional status.

2. Methodology

2.1. Subjects

The subjects were members of a female volleyball team, which was ranked in the national division. The team consisted of 15 members, 10 of which agreed to participate in the study. Five players refused to participate stating that their nutritional status was optimal. A written consent was obtained from all participating players. The age of the subjects ranged from 18 to 26 years. All were Caucasian and had been playing competitive volleyball for over 6 years. They trained 10-12 hours per week and their daily schedules included skill and strength training.

2.2. Questionnaire

The subjects completed a general history questionnaire, which was designed especially for the study in order to identify risk factors (medical, dietary and socioeconomic) related to the nutritional status of the subjects. The questionnaire was validated for Greek female athletes (pretested in a sample of Greek female athletes participating in different sports). It included 20 simple questions providing information on weight history, health status, appetite, living conditions, economic status, eating and drinking habits, drugs and supplements use, dieting, psychological status and menstrual cycle. Athletes were considered to be at risk for low nutritional status if they reported a particular risk factor on the general history questionnaire.

2.3. Anthropometric Measurements

Height was measured to the nearest 0.5 cm using a wall-mounted calibrated stadiometer (Ka We Measuring Instrument 44442). Weight was measured to the nearest 0.1 kg on a portable electronic beam scale (Philips Digital Bathroomscales HP 5320). Body mass index (BMI) was calculated as body weight / height^2. Body composition (fat mass and fat-free mass) was estimated via 2-site skinfold measurements (triceps and subscapular), using a Harpenden skinfold caliper and mid-upper-arm-circumference (MAC), using a flexible measuring tape according to Frisancho [10]. The same person took all measurements to the nearest 0.5 mm. Body fat mass was calculated from body density estimations according to Durnin and Womersley [8] and percent fat mass was estimated according to Siri [27]. Body fat-free mass was assessed from mid-upper-arm-muscle circumference (MAMC), which was calculated according to Frisancho from measurements of the mid-upper-arm-circumference (MAC) and triceps skinfolds [10].Anthropometric assessment was based on data for healthy American populations and used the guidelines for interpreting the age/sex percentile values for anthropometric indices proposed by Frisancho [10].

2.4. Dietary Assessment

Energy and nutrient intakes were determined from 7-day food records. Participants were given detailed instructions on how to complete food records during a group educational session, with measuring utensils and food models as instructional tools. Food records were completed during a 7-day recording period, at the time of food intake, after self-estimation of portion size according to instructions. Diet records were analyzed using Nutrition software (Version 6.4, 1998, ESHA Research). The nutrient database used, included data derived from analyses of traditional meal recopies, taken from a widely used Greek cookery book. Nutrient intake analysis did not include nutrient supplements, because the aim of the study was to evaluate the adequacy of dietary intake. Any additional use of supplements was however recorded and assessed in cases where risk to nutritional status was detected.

Total daily Energy Expenditure was estimated from calculations of Basal Metabolic Rate according to Schofield [26] and the energy expended in various daily activities including training, according to their duration and energy cost [4, 7].

Energy costs of individual physical activities were estimated from 7-day, self reported physical activity records, which were completed and collected at the same time as food records. Information collected regarding training included duration, type and intensity of training.

Nutrient intakes were assessed according to the current nutritional recommendations for athletes [7, 13–15, 17, 21].

3. Biochemical assessment

Fasting blood samples, drawn during the week of food and physical activity recording, were used for analyses. Hemoglobin and hematocrit levels and serum levels of albumin, iron, Total Iron Binding Capacity (TIBC), total cholesterol, HDL-cholesterol, LDL-cholesterol and triglycerides were assayed by a Clinical laboratory belonging to the Greek National Health System. The coefficient of variation (C.V.) of all assay methods was <5 % according to the quality control procedures of the laboratory involved. Athletes with low nutritional status were those who had values outside the reference range used by the laboratory.

4. Results

Risk factors for low nutritional status identified in the Greek team of female volleyball players included poor weight control, poor appetite, food avoidance, anemia, smoking, alcohol consumption, low blood pressure and constipation (Table 1). None of the athletes reported to be following special nutritional advice relating to health and optimum performance. All ten subjects had normal menstrual cycles and none reported being on a special diet or to be using medication. One athlete used iron and calcium supplements and two athletes were smokers and alcohol consumers. Three athletes reported recent weight gain and two athletes reported recent weight loss. Three athletes reported having anemia whereas another reported having low blood pressure. One player reported suffering from constipation. Half of the athletes reported poor appetite and food avoidance. One athlete avoided meat, another avoided vegetables and half of the athletes avoided pulses.

The age of athletes ranged from 18 to 26 years (Table 2). Mean height, weight and body mass index (BMI) were 1.75 ± 0.05 m (range 1.68 – 1.88 m), 63 ± 7 kg (range 54 – 79 kg) and 20.5 ± 1.7 kg/m^2 (range 18.2 – 22.7 kg/m^2) respectively. Eight athletes were tall (>/= 95th percentile) one was of above average height (85th percentile) and another athlete was of average height (75th – 85th percentile). Two athletes had weights above average (85th – 95th percentile) and eight athletes had average weights (25th – 75th percentile). Six athletes had average values for body mass index (25th – 75th percentile)

Nutritional Risk Factor	No of athletes at risk for low status
Menstrual cycle	0
Anemia	3
Constipation	1
Low Blood pressure	1
Drug therapy	0
Weight history	5
Alcohol consumption	2
Smoking	2
Low appetite	5
Food avoidance	5
Special Diet	0

TABLE 1: Nutritional Risk Factors for female volleyball players studied.

	Mean ± SD	Reference limits	No of athletes with low status	Range of values
Age (y)	22 ± 2	n.a.	n.a.	18 – 26
Height (m)	1.75 ± 0.05	1.52 – 1.74*	–	1.68 – 1.88
Weight (kg)	63 ± 7	46 – 84*	–	54 – 79
BMI (kg/m^2)	20.5 ± 1.7	17.7 – 32.1*	–	18.2 – 22.7
Body fat (%)	27 ± 7	17 – 35 **	–	21 – 32
MAMC (mm)	214 ± 22	183 – 249*	1	180 – 254

TABLE 2: Anthropometric characteristics of female volleyball players studied. * Reference limits are the 5th and 95th percentile values for age and sex ( ). **Upper reference limit is the 85th percentile value for age and sex ( ).

while four athletes had values below average (5th – 15th percentile). Mean body fat percentage was 27 ± 7 (range 21 – 32) and the mean value for MAMC was 214 ± 22 mm (range 180 – 254 mm). All athletes had average fat mass (15th – 75th percentile), seven athletes had average muscle mass (25th – 75th percentile), one athlete had low muscle status – wasted (<5th percentile) and two athletes had high muscle status – good nutrition (above 95th percentile). Three athletes with below average body mass index had average fat and muscle mass while the fourth athlete had more fat mass than the others and lower muscle mass-wasted.

Daily mean intakes of energy and nutrients and number of athletes with low intakes are shown in Table 3. Mean energy intake (EI) was 1861 ± 337 kcal/d (range 1450 – 2597 kcal/d) while mean energy expenditure (EE) was 2060 ± 234 kcal/d (range 1785 – 2576 kcal/d); the mean daily physical activity level (PAL) was 1.5. Daily energy intakes of five athletes were reported to be below 1800 kcal/d. Seven athletes appeared to be in negative energy balance (EI / EE < 1) while three athletes appeared to be in positive energy balance (EI / EE > 1).

Mean energy intake per kg of body weight was 30 ± 7 kcal/kg/d (range 21 - 43 kcal/kg/d) and seven athletes might be at risk for low energy status required for anaerobic/aerobic exercise according to their reported energy intakes which were below recommended levels for athletes. Only one athlete reported a level of energy intake above 41 kcal/kg/d, which is a minimum level for anaerobic/aerobic exercise.

The contribution of protein, fat and carbohydrate to total energy intake was 13 ± 3 % (range 7 - 17 %), 39 ± 6 % (range 30 - 46 %), and 48 ± 7 % (range 38 - 54 %) respectively. Eight athletes reported high fat intake, above recommendations for health, which was assessed as a possible nutritional risk. Mean protein intake per kg of body weight was 1.0 ± 0.3 g/kg/d (range 0.4 – 1.6 g/kg/d) while seven athletes might have been at risk for low protein status since they reported protein intakes below the recommended level for aerobic/anaerobic sports. Mean carbohydrate intake per kg of body weight was 3.8 ± 0.9 g/kg/d (range 2.1 - 6.1 g/kg/d) and the reported carbohydrate intakes were below recommendations in nine athletes.

Six athletes had low intakes of vitamin C with mean intake of 66 ± 35 mg/d (range 23 – 122 mg/d). Mean intake of vitamin B12 was 3.8 ± 3.9 μg/d (range 1.0 – 13.4 μg/d) and six athletes also had intakes below recommendations. Niacin mean level of intake was 22 ± 18 mg/d (range 6 – 74 mg/d) with three athletes recording low levels. None of the athletes had an adequate intake of vitamin D (range 0.3 – 1.2 μg/d), vitamin E (range 0.9 – 5.4 mg/d), vitamin B6 (range of intakes 0.3 – 0.9 mg/d) and folate (range 65 – 271 μg/d). Only two athletes had adequate vitamin A intakes (range 175 – 2756 μg/d) while eight athletes had intakes in the range 175 - 659 μg/d well below recommendations. Two athletes had adequate B1 intakes (range of intakes 0.3 – 1.3 mg/d) and three had adequate B2 intakes (range 0.2 – 1.6 mg/d). Only one athlete had an adequate intake of iron from her diet (25 mg/d) and this athlete also had an adequate intake of calcium, when the calcium supplement she was using was taken into consideration. Only one athlete had an adequate intake of calcium from her diet (1400 mg/d).

All mean values of the biochemical indices studied and the number of players with low status are shown in Table 4. One athlete had low hemoglobin and three athletes had low serum iron and low transferrin saturation. Low iron and low transferrin saturation are indices of low iron stores while low hemoglobin is an index of more advanced deficiency of iron. All athletes had adequate protein status as shown by serum albumin levels. All athletes had normal levels of total cholesterol, HDL-cholesterol, LDL-cholesterol and triglycerides, showing normal risk to cardiovascular disease, except one athlete who might have slightly increased risk, indicated by slightly elevated levels of total cholesterol and LDL-cholesterol (204 mg/dl and 153 mg/dl respectively).

	Mean ± SD	Recommended values *	No of athletes at risk for low nutritional status	Range of reported values
Energy intake (kcal/d)	1861 ± 337	2060 ± 234**	7	1450 - 2597
Energy intake (kcal/kg/d)	30 ± 7	37 - 41	7	21 - 43
Carbohydrate intake (g/d)	234 ± 50			167 - 366
Carbohydrate intake (g/kg/d)	3.8 ± 0.9	5.0 - 10.0	9	2.1 - 6.1
% energy from carbohydrate	48 ± 7			38 - 54
Protein intake(g/d)	61 ± 19			26 - 95
Protein intake (g/kg/d)	1.0 ± 0.3	1.2 - 2.0	7	0.4 - 1.6
% of energy from protein	13 ± 3			7 - 17
Fat intake (g/d)	80 ± 20			48 - 116
% of energy from fat	39 ± 6	20 - 30	8	30 - 46
Vitamin A intake(μg)	825 ± 922	1000	8	175 - 2756
Vitamin D intake (μg)	0.7 ± 0.3	10	10	0.3 - 1.2
Vitamin E intake(mg)	2.7 ± 1.3	10	10	0.9 - 5.4
Vitamin C intake(mg)	66 ± 35	65	6	23 - 122
Vitamin B1 intake(mg)	0.7 ± 0.2	1.0	8	0.3 - 1.3
Vitamin B2 intake(mg)	0.8 ± 0.4	1.0	7	0.2 - 1.6
Vitamin B6 intake(mg)	0.6 ± 0.2	1.2	10	0.3 - 0.9
Vitamin B12 intake(μg)	3.8 ± 3.9	2.4	6	1.0 - 13.4
Niacin intake(mg)	22 ± 18	14	3	6 - 74
Folate intake (μg)	137 ± 57	400	10	65 - 271
Iron intake (mg) ***	10 ± 5	18	9	5.7 - 25.2
Calcium intake (mg) ***	688 ± 349	1300	9	249 - 1400

TABLE 3: Energy and nutrient intakes of female volleyball players studied. *Recommended Dietary Allowances or Dietary Reference Intakes (9, 15, 16, 17, 25, 26). **This is the reported level of Mean Energy Expenditure. ***Mineral supplements were not included in the analysis.

5. Discussion

Athletes are generally considered to be at risk for low nutritional status because of the extra demand for energy and nutrients imposed by the increased physical activity involved in daily training and competition, unless their energy and nutrient intakes are adequately increased.

Self-reported physical activity records collected in the present study showed a mean daily level of physical activity close to the levels expected for sedentary females and lower than the levels of physical activity derived from DLW energy expenditure

Index	Mean ± SD	Reference range*	No of athletes with low status	Range of assayed values
Hematocrit (%)	39 ± 2	36 - 47	0	37 - 41
Hemoglobin (g/dl)	12.7 ± 1.2	12 - 16	1	11 - 15
Serum iron (μg/dl)	60 ± 17	60 - 145	3	36 - 86
Serum TIBC (μg/dl)	297 ± 29	250 - 350	0	254 - 340
Transferin saturation (%)	20 ± 5	>16	3	12 - 27
Serum albumin (g/dl)	4.0 ± 2	3.5 - 4.5	0	3.6 - 4.4
Serum total cholesterol (mg/dl)	159 ± 31	100 - 200	1**	109 - 204
Serum HDL cholesterol (mg/dl)	47 ± 8	35 - 55	0	38 - 60
Serum LDL cholesterol (mg/dl)	98 ± 32	<150	1**	51 - 153
Serum triglycerides (mg/dl)	66 ± 19	30 - 220	0	38 - 102

TABLE 4: Biochemical indices for female volleyball players studied. *Reference range used by the laboratory, which carried out the tests. ** Low status indicates high risk for cardiovascular disease.

studies of athletes [4]. Apparently our athletes either under-reported their levels of physical activity due to systematic errors in recording despite instructions, or had lower daily physical activity levels than other athletes. One generally assumes that training increases the daily level of physical activity in all athletes, and that it has no effect on the level of physical activity during time not spent in exercise. Athletes usually spend variable lengths of time to rest after strenuous training, depending on their nutritional status and time allowances of their daily schedule.

Based on physical activity records, energy expenditure of seven athletes in the present study was not matched by their reported energy intakes. These athletes appeared to be in negative energy balance during the week of data collection. Discrepancies between reported energy intakes and energy requirements in female athletes have been reported in the literature, and might indicate under-reporting [4, 9]. These discrepancies might not correspond to habitual dietary intakes and long-term nutritional status. The weight changes reported by five athletes in this study indicate a long-term energy imbalance at least in these athletes. Reported energy imbalances however do not correspond to reported weight changes or anthropometric nutrition indexes of the athletes concerned. This suggests that the reported dietary data might not reflect long term nutrition of the athletes, either because of changes in dietary habits during the period of data collection or under-reporting of food intake by some athletes [4]. Two athletes in the present study were suspect for under-reporting (they had a low ratio of EI / EE of 0.7). It is worth noting that these athletes had high muscle status, indicating adequate habitual dietary intake. These athletes obviously did not report habitual dietary intake, probably led by misconceptions regarding appropriate nutrition and body composition of athletes.

The mean energy intake of the team (30 ± 7 kcal/kg/d) was below the levels reported by American female athletes [2] but similar to the levels reported by Greek female athletes [9, 20]. Mean protein intake in the present study (1.0 ± 0.3 g/kg/d) was similar to the level reported by Greek female volleyball players [20] but lower than the level reported by Greek female aquatic athletes [9]. Mean carbohydrate intake in the present study (3.8 ± 0.9 g/kg/d) was similar to the levels reported by Greek female volleyball and aquatic athletes [9, 20]. Mean protein and carbohydrate intakes were lower than those reported by American female volleyball and soccer players [2, 18]. Seven players were at risk for low protein status according to their reported protein intakes (Table 3). If the reported low intakes of energy and protein reflect habitual intakes, they might lead to failure to sustain desirable muscle mass. Muscle mass status was average for most athletes in our study, at similar levels to sedentary individuals. One athlete, who reported avoiding meat and pulses, had significantly low muscle mass status indicating muscle wasting. Her reported levels of energy and protein intakes were, however, similar to the mean values of the team. Serum levels of albumin show long-term changes in protein status and are insensitive to short-term changes, due to the relatively long half-life (14 – 20 days) of albumin. Short- term changes due to stress and short-term dietary changes cannot influence serum albumin levels.

Adequate carbohydrate intakes are essential for maintaining athletic performance. The recommended levels for carbohydrate intakes for high intensity endurance male athletes are 5 – 10 g/kg/d respectively [21].

Nine athletes in the present study reported carbohydrate intakes below the recommended level suggesting that they were at risk for low performance. Low carbohydrate intakes may result in low glycogen stores and inability of the athlete to sustain high intensity energy demands.

Mean fat intake was similar to the intake reported by Greek female volleyball players [20], higher than that reported by Greek female aquatic athletes and American female volleyball athletes [2, 9] and higher than the recommended levels for optimum health [7, 22]. Eight athletes had fat intakes higher than 30 % of total energy intake. High fat intake might be related to poor weight control, which was reported by five athletes. The long-term negative effects of high fat diets on health are well known. One athlete faced increased risk for cardiovascular disease indicated by slightly elevated levels of total and LDL-cholesterol. Athletes should follow the general recommendations for health regarding fat intake. Typically diets containing 20-25 % energy from fat have been recommended to facilitate adequate carbohydrate intake and to assist in weight management where necessary [21].

Mean micronutrient intakes were similar to those reported by Greek female volleyball players [20] and lower than the intakes reported by Greek female aquatic athletes (Farajian et al. 004) and American female volleyball and soccer players [2, 18].

Most athletes reported low intakes of antioxidant vitamins. Although a well-trained athlete may have a more developed endogenous antioxidant system than a sedentary person, athletes should meet the general recommendations for health [21].

An inadequate intake of antioxidant vitamins could place athletes at greater risk for damage resulting from oxidative stresses and result in slower recovery from exercise-induced damage.

The reported intakes of the B-complex vitamins were also low for most athletes with the exception of niacin. Taking into account that exercise may slightly increase the need for these vitamins, low intakes may impair energy production during exercise, production of red cells, protein synthesis and tissue repair and maintenance [21].

Low calcium and iron dietary intakes were reported by nine athletes. One athlete used iron supplementation when her dietary intake was already adequate. The same athlete managed to meet recommendations for calcium intake by using calcium supplementation. Inadequate calcium intake found in eight athletes increases the risk for low mineral density and stress fractures [29].

Low iron intake is one of the causes for low iron status. Iron deficiency anemia was diagnosed in one athlete and iron depletion (low iron stores) was found in three athletes according to biochemical indices (Table 4). All three athletes reported avoiding pulses, a very important food source for iron in many areas and diets [24]. Iron depletion is one of the most prevalent nutrient deficiencies, mostly observed in female athletes. No significant impact of iron depletion on exercise performance has been observed, but iron deficiency anemia as a result of iron depletion can certainly affect exercise performance negatively [21]. Early detection and supplementation may improve performance [6].

The reported low energy intake of most athletes in the present study might partially explain their low intake of micronutrients. Beside sufficient energy intake however, a large variety of foods consumed in appropriate amounts as defined by the Food Pyramids is essential to ensure adequate macronutrient and micronutrient intake.

The anthropometric assessment in the present study showed that mean height, weight and body mass index was similar to Greek and American female volleyball players [2, 20]. Mean body fat however was above the level reported for female athletes participating in similar sports and the levels reported for American female volleyball players [2, 21]. The estimated minimal level of body fat compatible with health is 12 % for females. However, optimal body fat percentages for an individual athlete may be much higher than this minimum and should be determined on an individual basis [21]. It should be born in mind however that reduced body fat levels could help volleyball players optimize speed, agility and jumping ability [5].

Mid-upper-arm muscle-circumference can be used to assess total muscle mass and is frequently used for this purpose in field surveys. It can also be used to assess large changes in total body muscle mass, but is insensitive to small changes. Reduction in MAMC is indicative of muscle degradation in order to provide essential amino acids and is seen in chronic dietary deficiency of protein and energy [10].

The low muscle status that was diagnosed in one athlete might be interpreted as a result of chronic dietary deficiency of protein and energy. Only two athletes in the present study were assessed, according to their muscle mass, as having high muscle status- good nutrition, as would be expected for athletes engaged in sports that emphasize strength. Muscle mass estimations corresponding to female athletes, were not found in the literature for comparison. Because of possible errors associated with body composition assessment methods (validity of prediction equations used), body composition values should be interpreted with caution.

6. Conclusion

Reported energy, protein and carbohydrate intakes of most volleyball players in the present study were at levels lower than recommended. Under-reporting might have affected the dietary assessment of some players but poor weight control, low muscle status and low iron status in some players, indicate long-term energy and nutrient imbalances. High fat intake was probably related to poor weight control and increased risk for cardiovascular disease. Low micronutrient intake was partly due to low energy intake and partly to avoidance of nutrient dense foods. Low protein status was assessed in one athlete, (low muscle mass, low dietary intakes of energy and protein, and avoidance of meat and pulses), low iron status was assessed in three athletes, (low iron stores, low intake of iron, and avoidance of pulses) and elevated risk for cardiovascular disease was assessed in one athlete, (high serum cholesterol, high serum LDL-cholesterol and high intake of dietary fat). There is an urgent need for nutrition counseling of athletes, based on individual needs for optimum health and performance.

7. Conflict of Interests

The authors declare that there is no conflict of interests regarding the publication of this paper.

8. Acknowledgment

We would like to express our sincere thanks towards Professor Kalliopi Kleftouri for her contribution to the paper.

References

[1] C. P. Arun, "Drive for leanness, anorexia nervosa, and overactivity: The missing link," *Annals of the New York Academy of Sciences*, vol. 1148, pp. 526–529, 2008.

[2] K. A. Beals, "Eating behaviors, nutritional status, and menstrual function in elite female adolescent volleyball players," *Journal of the American Dietetic Association*, vol. 102, no. 9, pp. 1293–1296, 2002.

[3] J. E. Benson, Y. Allemann, G. E. Theintz, and H. Howald, "Eating problems and calorie intake levels in Swiss adolescent athletes," *International Journal of Sports Medicine*, vol. 11, no. 4, pp. 249–252, 1990.

[4] A. E. Black, "Dietary assessment for sports dietetics," *Nutrition Bulletin*, vol. 26, no. 1, pp. 29–42, 2001.

[5] GB. Carey, "Nutrition: the winning diet," in *Science of Coaching Volleyball*, C. McGown, Ed., pp. 130–160, Human Kinetics, Champaign, IL, 1994.

[6] D. M. DellaValle, "Iron Supplementation for Female Athletes," *Current Sports Medicine Reports*, vol. 12, no. 4, pp. 234–239, 2013.

[7] M. Wiseman, "The COMA Report: Dietary Reference Values for Food Energy and Nutrients for the United Kingdom," *British Food Journal*, vol. 94, no. 3, pp. 7–9, 1992.

[8] J. V. Durnin and J. Womersley, "Body fat assessed from total body density and its estimation from skinfold thickness: measurements on 481 men and women aged from 16 to 72 years," *British Journal of Nutrition*, vol. 32, no. 1, pp. 77–97, 1974.

[9] P. Farajian, S. A. Kavouras, M. Yannakoulia, and L. S. Sidossis, "Dietary intake and nutritional practices of elite Grek aquatic athletes," *International Journal of Sport Nutrition and Exercise Metabolism*, vol. 14, no. 5, pp. 574–585, 2004.

[10] A. Frisancho, *Anthropometric Standards for the Assessment of Growth and Nutritional Status*, University of Michigan Press, Ann Arbor, MI, 1990.

[11] J. C. Gibson, L. Stuart-Hill, S. Martin, and C. Gaul, "Nutrition status of junior elite canadian female soccer athletes," *International Journal of Sport Nutrition and Exercise Metabolism*, vol. 21, no. 6, pp. 507–514, 2011.

[12] M. N. Hassapidou and A. Manstrantoni, "Dietary intakes of elite female athletes in Greece," *Journal of Human Nutrition and Dietetics*, vol. 14, no. 5, pp. 391–396, 2001.

[13] Board., *Dietary Reference Intakes for Calcium, Phosphorous, Magnesium, Vitamin D, and Fluoride. Washington DC*, National Academy Press, Institute of Medicine, Food and Nutrition, Washington DC, 1997.

[14] *Dietary Reference Intakes for Thiamin, Riboflavin, Niacin, Vitamin B6, Folate, Vitamin B12, Pantothenic Acid, Biotin, and Choline*, National Academies Press, Washington, D.C., 1998.

[15] A. Bendich, "Dietary reference intakes for vitamin C, vitamin E, selenium, and carotenoids institute of medicine washington, DC: National Academy Press, 2000 ISBN: 0-309-06935-1," *Nutrition*, vol. 17, no. 4, p. 364, 2001.

[16] M. Jette, "Guide for anthropometric classification of Canadian adults for use in nutritional assessment. Health and Welfare," *Guide for anthropometric classification of Canadian adults for use in nutritional assessment. Health and Welfare*, 1981.

[17] R. J. Maughan and L. M. Burke, "Practical Nutritional Recommendations for the Athlete," in *Sports Nutrition: More Than Just Calories – Triggers for Adaptation*, vol. 69 of *Nestlé Nutrition Institute Workshop Series*, pp. 131–149, Karger, Basel, 2012.

[18] M. C. Mullinix, S. S. Jonnalagadda, C. A. Rosenbloom, W. R. Thompson, and J. R. Kicklighter, "Dietary intake of female U.S. soccer players," *Nutrition Research*, vol. 23, no. 5, pp. 585–593, 2003.

[19] J. Nutter, "Seasonal changes in female athletes diets," *Int J Sport Nutr*, vol. 12, p. S35, 1991.

[20] S. K. Papadopoulou, S. D. Papadopoulou, and G. K. Gallos, "Macro- and micro-nutrient intake of adolescent Greek female volleyball players," *International Journal of Sport Nutrition*, vol. 12, no. 1, pp. 73–80, 2002.

[21] "Position of the American Dietetic Association, Dietitians of Canada, and the American College of Sports Medicine," *Journal of the American Dietetic Association*, vol. 100, no. 12, pp. 1543–1556, 2000.

[22] *Recommended Dietary Allowances, 10th*, National Academies Press, Washington, D.C., 1989.

[23] J. L. Reed, M. J. De Souza, J. M. Kindler, and N. I. Williams, "Nutritional practices associated with low energy availability in Division I female soccer players," *Journal of Sports Sciences*, vol. 32, no. 16, pp. 1499–1509, 2014.

[24] A. C. Roba, K. Gabriel-Micheal, G. A. Zello, J. Jaffe, S. J. Whiting, and C. J. Henry, "A Low Pulse Food Intake May Contribute to the Poor Nutritional Status and Low Dietary Intakes of Adolescent Girls in Rural Southern Ethiopia," *Ecology of Food and Nutrition*, vol. 54, no. 3, pp. 240–254, 2015.

[25] A. E. Scates, Winning Volleyball. Dubuque IA: Brown & Benchmark, 1993.

[26] W. N. Schofield, "Predicting basal metabolic rate, new standards and review of previous work," *Human Nutrition: Clinical Nutrition*, vol. 39, supplement 1, pp. 5–41, 1985.

[27] W. E. Siri, "Body composition from fluid spaces and density: Analysis of methods," in *Techniques for Measuring Body Composition*, pp. 223–244, National Academy of Sciences, National Research Council, Washington, 1961.

[28] J. Sundgot-Borgen, "Risk and trigger factors for the development of eating disorders in female elite athletes," *Medicine & Science in Sports & Exercise*, vol. 26, no. 4, pp. 414–419, 1994.

[29] L. Wentz, P.-Y. Liu, J. Z. Ilich, and E. M. Haymes, "Dietary and training predictors of stress fractures in female runners," *International Journal of Sport Nutrition and Exercise Metabolism*, vol. 22, no. 5, pp. 374–382, 2012.

[30] G. Wollenberg, L. H. Shriver, and G. E. Gates, "Comparison of disordered eating symptoms and emotion regulation difficulties between female college athletes and non-athletes," *Eating Behaviors*, vol. 18, pp. 1–6, 2015.

[31] J. Zapolska, K. Witczak, and A. Manczuk, "Assessment of nutrition, supplementation and body composition parameters on the example of professional volleyball players. Rocz Panstw Zakl Hig," in *Ma□czuk A*, vol. 65(3), pp. 235–242, 2014.

2

Assessment of Body Composition, Endurance and Nutrient Intakes among Females Team Players in Sports Club

Amita Attlee[1,2], Shaimaa S. Altunaiji[1], Mariam Muayyad[1], Zainab Ali[1], Mona Hashim[1,2], and Reyad S. Obaid[1,2]

[1]Department of Clinical Nutrition and Dietetics, College of Health Sciences, University of Sharjah, Sharjah, UAE
[2]Research Institute of Medical and Health Sciences, University of Sharjah, Sharjah, UAE

Corresponding Author: Amita Attlee; email: aattlee@sharjah.ac.ae

Abstract

Aim: The aim of the study was to assess the body composition, endurance level and usual nutrient intakes in female players representing a Sports Club in Sharjah, United Arab Emirates.

Materials and Methods: Twenty-six adult female players aged between 15-24 years were selected from three different teams (basketball = 12, tennis = 4, volleyball = 10) using convenience sampling technique. All participants were assessed for body composition through bioelectrical impedance method, endurance level using step test and nutrient intakes using 24-hour recall method. Significant differences ($P < 0.05$) were determined among the three teams in relation to body composition, endurance levels and nutrient intakes.

Results: Body composition of players in three sports was significantly different in terms of body mass index, body fat mass, and percentage body fat and fitness scores. Tennis players had significantly higher body fat mass (28.5 ± 8.2 kg) and percent body fat (41 ± 7%) in contrast to that in basketball players (body fat mass: 19.2 ± 10.5 kg; percent body fat: 30.6 ± 7.9%) and tennis players (body fat mass: 13 ± 4.2 kg; percent body fat: 26.5 ± 6.5%), respectively. On the other hand, volleyball players had significantly higher fitness score (72.2 ± 3.5) as compared to basketball players (71 ± 6.7), and tennis players (63 ± 8.2).

On an average, volleyball players scored "very good" endurance level in contrast to "good" scores in basketball and tennis team players. However, this difference was not statistically significant.

The average intakes of all nutrients including energy, protein, vitamins and minerals were below the recommended intakes among players of all sports teams.

Conclusions: Body composition and endurance level differ with the type of sports. Volleyball team players had the lowest BMI, body fat mass as well as percent body fat and highest fitness score and endurance level. However, the overall nutrient intakes of the female players representing the three teams were less than the recommended allowances for highly active women and did not differ with the type of sports played.

Keywords: Body composition, endurance, nutrient intake, sports team players

1. Introduction

Sport clubs have become an integral part of the social infra-structure of almost every nation, offering organized sports activities, thereby building skills and promoting health of the individuals [11]. Training through organized sports enables all the game players to develop comprehensive skills including physical, technical, mental, and tactical abilities [6]. The world's popular sports like tennis, basketball and volleyball also require varying levels of competence, high level of technical and tactical skills as well as suitable anthropometric characteristics for successful participation [6].

Anthropometric measurements, parameters of the body composition such as body fat, fat-free mass (FFM) and somatotype components are often used to evaluate these physical abilities [20]. Somatic traits and body composition are influenced by the training and type of sport pursued [2].

Lean body mass compared to total body weight is closely related to physiological parameters such as oxygen consumption, cardiac output, vital capacity, etc. [19]. Basketball and volleyball players are typically taller than the players of other games [20]. Moreover, mean body height and weight, body fat as well as fat free mass of basketball players were found to be higher than those of volleyball players [6].

Female sports players need to be well conditioned to meet the intense demands of the game. Endurance training of moderate to high intensity is crucial for achieving a higher level of performance of female sports players [17]. They must be quick to move, and have strength and power. The functional performance of any complex chain of torque transfers, that is, serve or ground strokes in tennis depends on several factors including technique, flexibility, muscle strength, speed, and power [18].

Sports players undergo special nutrient demands because of enhanced metabolic process developed through extensive exercise; repetitive cycle of food deprivation might lead to a nutritionally undesirable state and dehydration problems [8]. Female sports players need to consume enough energy and appropriate nutrition to maintain their competitive edge for training and competition. Further, nutritional problems related to micronutrients leads to substandard training and impaired performance [5].

Energy and nutrients intake among athletes are influenced by many factors; type of activity, intensity and duration in addition to body composition of the athletes. Carbohydrates are the master fuel for these athletes, its needs are similar among most types, varying between 6–10 g carbohydrates /kg body weight per day, accounting for 50–65% of total daily calories. Likewise, protein requirements vary with the type of activity and are estimated to be 1.2 to 1.4 g/kg body weight, 1.2–2.0 g/kg per day for endurance and team sports respectively comprising of about 15–20% total calories. Dietary composition of fat is a contribution of ~ 20–35% of total calories, the majority should be in the form of unsaturated fats [9].

In spite of the fact that nutrition is an influential determinant of athletics performance, female athletes often show poor dietary behavior that can affect their successful physical performance [7]. The diets of female athletes have been found to be inadequate in the consumption of carbohydrates and protein, as well as micronutrients like vitamin E, magnesium, folate, and zinc [10].

Female sports are gaining impetus in the United Arab Emirates (UAE), especially among the youth. Ladies sports clubs have been established to manage and develop the local talent and empower women with the knowledge and skills of different sports. Due to the lack of evidence on the physical status of the female sports players in the UAE, the present study was designed to assess the body composition, level of endurance and nutrient intakes among adult female players representing sports teams in s sports club.

2. Materials and Methods

A cross-sectional research design was adopted. Adult females representing the sport teams at Sharjah Ladies Club were assessed. The teams were coached by highly efficient and qualified trainers in order to improve the level of the athletes to reach international tournaments.

2.1. Sample

Twenty-six (26) adult female sports team members representing Sharjah Ladies Club including twelve (12) from basketball team, ten (10) from volleyball team and four (4) from tennis teams were selected.

All the players in the current study were members of competitive teams that contest for top honors in local, Arab and international championships. All players were informed about the aim of the study and signed a written consent before the data collection. The study was approved by the Department Research Committee, Clinical Nutrition and Dietetics department, College of Health Sciences, University of Sharjah. A pre-tested, semi-coded interview schedule was formulated and administrated on the sports team players.

2.2. Body Composition

It was assessed by using Bioelectrical Impedance Analysis (BIA) (Biospace Co. Ltd., Model: Inbody 230, Korea). The players were informed in advance about the protocol for measuring their body compositions. They were instructed to restrict physical exercise at least 1 day prior to the test. None of the players were pregnant or had metal implants. The test was performed in the morning after 10-12 hours of overnight fasting. Each player was made to stand on body composition analysis machine with the light clothing and no socks, stockings or metals on the body. It was ensured that each player stood on the machine in proper posture: bare feet maintaining contact with the electrodes and thumbs of the arms placed on the electrode pads on the top surface of the handle. The data were entered for each player's identification, age, height and sex by the researcher. Height was measured by Harpenden stadiometer using the following technique [13]. Weight, total body water (TBW), body fat mass, muscle mass, body mass index (BMI), percent body fat (%BF), basal metabolic rate (BMR), and fitness score were determined with the BIA machine for body composition.

2.3. Endurance

Modified Canadian Aerobic Fitness Test (mCAFT) was used to measure the level of endurance [12]. mCAFT is used as a multistage step test to assess sub-maximal exercise capacity. Each player was asked to perform a series of stepping sequences on a 20.3 cm step in time with a musical cadence. Starting stage or stepping sequence was determined according to the subject's age. Each stage lasted for 3 minutes and progressively became more challenging. To begin with, the resting blood pressure and resting heart rate of each player were measured. At the end of each stage, heart rate was measured, if it was below the 85% of predicted maximum heart rate, the player was allowed to proceed and the next stage started. On the other hand, the player was not allowed to move to higher stage if her heart rate reached above 85% of predicted maximum heart rate or any discomfort such as nausea, extreme leg pain, chest pain, or any adverse symptom was experienced. At the end of all stages, blood pressure and heart rate at four minutes post exercise were measured. An oxygen uptake value for the final stepping stage was taken from the Canadian Standardized Test of Fitness Operations Manual [7].

Originally, physical fitness is evaluated according to 5 categories (Need Improvement, Fair, Good, Very good and Excellent). However, in the present study, these were merged into 3 categories (Need Improvement, Good and Very Good) to overcome the effect of small sample size.

2.4. Nutrient Intakes

Nutrient intakes were estimated from the 24-hour dietary recall method. This method was preferred over the other dietary assessment methods because of its advantages. It involves little respondent burden; because of the immediacy of the recall period, respondents are able to recall most of their dietary intake. Also, those who agree to give 24-hour dietary recalls are more likely to be representative of the population than are those who agree to keep food records. In contrast to record methods, dietary recalls occur after the food has been consumed, so there is less potential for the assessment method to interfere with dietary behavior [21].

Each player was asked to recall in detail all the food items and drinks consumed during period of time in the last 24-hours (previous day). The researchers recorded this information for later coding and analysis [13]. Nutrient intakes were calculated and compared with the dietary reference intakes (DRIs) for their age and sex through ESHA Food Processor Software (ESHAPortSQL 2012). Thirteen nutrients have been reported, namely, energy, protein, thiamin, riboflavin, niacin, vitamin B_6, vitamin B_{12}, vitamin A, folate, vitamin C, calcium, magnesium, iron and zinc and compared with the dietary reference intakes (DRIs) was estimated [22].

2.5. Statistical Analysis

The data was subjected to descriptive statistics using Statistical Package for the Social Sciences SPSS 17 Version program (SPSS, USA). Body composition, endurance and nutrient intakes variables were expressed as means and standard deviations. One-way ANOVA test was used to determine if significant differences ($p < 0.05$) existed among the three teams in relation to body composition variables and nutrient intake. Chi square test was used to determine the association in endurance level variables among the players from different sport teams. When there was a significance difference variable, a post hoc test (Least Square Difference) was used to identify specific differences among the teams.

3. Results

The average age of the players was 19.8 years ranging between 18-24 years. Majority of the players were Emirati nationals (n = 20) and the rest were expatriates from other countries (n = 6).

3.1. Body Composition

The means and standard deviations of body composition for the players in three sports teams are presented in Table 1. In addition, the critical differences in their body composition are depicted in Table 2. As evident, the heights of the players ranged from 151-185 cm with the mean height of basketball players being relatively higher than the tennis and volleyball players. However, this difference was not statistically significant. Similarly, the basketball players weighed heavier (57 ± 8.2 kg) as compared to tennis players (52.6 ± 3.2 kg) and volleyball players (52 ± 4.6 kg) with no significant differences among the teams.

BMI ranged from 17 kg/m^2 to 39 kg/m^2, average being 22 ± 0.9 kg/m^2 (Table 1). The tennis players had significantly higher BMI than the basketball and volleyball players. Specifically, this significant difference was observed between the BMI values of tennis and volleyball players (Table 2). According to WHO [23] classification, the average BMI indicated that the tennis players were overweight in contrast to the other teams who were found to be in the normal BMI category. Similar trend was evident in the body fat mass of the players in three sports with a significantly higher in tennis players (28.6 ± 8.2 kg) in contrast to basketball (22.6 ± 1.08) kg and volleyball players (13 ± 4.2 kg). Significant difference in fat mass existed between tennis and volleyball players. Further, tennis players had significantly higher %BF (40.9 ± 6.9 %) as compared to basketball (30.6 ± 7.9 %) as well as volleyball players (26.6 ± 6.5 %).

Fitness score of the female sports team players was 70.2 ± 0.4, on average (Table 1). Volleyball and basketball players had significantly higher fitness scores than the tennis players (72.2 ± 0.4; 71 ± 0.4; 63 ± 0.5, respectively).

3.2. Endurance

On an average, the female players in the three teams scored "good" level of endurance (Table 3). Volleyball players showed "very good" endurance that was relatively higher

Body composition	Total players (n = 26)	Basketball players (n = 12)	Tennis players (n = 4)	Volleyball players (n = 10)	P value
variables	(Mean ± SD)	(Mean ± SD)	(Mean ± SD)	(Mean ± SD)	
Height (cm)	160 ± 6.8	162.3 ± 8.4	158 ± 3.4	158.4 ± 5.2	0.335
Weight (kg)	54.6 ± 6.7	57.2 ± 8.2	52.6 ± 3.2	52.2 ± 4.6	0.182
BMI (kg/m^2)	22.2 ± 0.9	22.6 ± 1.08	27.5 ± 0.8	19.6 ± 0.47	0.018*
Percentage Body Fat (%)	30.6 ± 8.5	30.6 ± 7.9	40.9 ± 6.9	26.6 ± 6.5	0.011*
Body Fat Mass (kg)	18.4 ± 9.5	19.2 ± 10.5	28.6 ± 8.2	13.3 ± 4.2	0.017*
Muscle Mass (kg)	20.9 ± 3.4	22 ± 4.5	21.7 ± 1.6	19.3 ± 1.2	0.156
Total Body Water (kg)	28.4 ± 4.2	29.8 ± 5.6	29.4 ± 2.07	26.3 ± 1.5	0.144
Basal Metabolic Rate (kcal)	1208 ± 125.3	1248.8 ± 165.7	1237 ± 61.7	1147 ± 46	0.148
Fitness Score	70.2± 0.4	71 ± 0.4	63 ± 0.5	72.2 ± 0.4	0.044*

TABLE 1: Body composition of female team players. * Significant at $P < 0.05$; SD: Standard deviation.

(456 ± 54.3) as compared to basketball (383 ± 84.6) and tennis (384 ± 51.2) players. However, the difference was not statistically significant.

3.3. Nutrient Intakes

Nutrient intakes of the female players are presented in Table 4. As evident, the results revealed that consumption levels of most of the nutrients were below the recommendations with no significant differences in nutrient intakes amongst the female players in the three sports teams.

4. Discussion

The present study highlighted the body composition, endurance as well as nutrient intakes among basketball, tennis and volleyball female players. Our findings were consistent with the results of Gaurav et al. [6]. They also reported that the basketball players were significantly taller than volleyball players. In addition, tennis players were

Body composition parameters			Mean Difference	Std. Error	P value
BMI (kg/m^2)	Basketball	X Volleyball	2.955	1.848	0.12
	Tennis	X Basketball	4.875	2.491	0.06
	Tennis	X Volleyball	7.830*	2.553	0.01
Body fat %	Basketball	X Volleyball	4.048	3.126 4.216 4.320	0.21 0.02 0.00
	Tennis	X Basketball	10.342* 14.290*		
	Tennis	X Volleyball			
Body Fat Mass (kg)	Basketball	X Volleyball	5.962	3.574	0.11
	Tennis	X Basketball	9.333	4.819	0.06
	Tennis	X Volleyball	15.295*	4.938	0.01
Fitness Score	Basketball	X Tennis	8.000*	3.438	0.03
	Volleyball	X Basketball	1.2	2.550 3.523	0.64
	Volleyball	X Tennis	9.200*		0.02

TABLE 2: Comparison of body composition among female team players (n = 26). * Significant at $p < 0.05$.

Sport Team	Endurance Score	Endurance Level		
	Mean ± SD	Need Improvement	Good	Very Good
		350 or less – 377	378 – 419	420 - 472 or more
		N (%)	N (%)	N (%)
Basketball	383± 84.6	4 (33%)	4 (33%)	4 (33%)
Tennis	384 ± 51.2	2 (50%)	1 (25%)	1 (25%)
Volleyball	456 ± 54.3	1 (10%)	0	9 (90%)
Total	412 ± 76.1	7 (27%)	5 (19%)	14 (54%)

TABLE 3: Endurance level of female players in sports teams (n = 26).

Nutrient	Total	Basketball players (Mean ± SD)	Tennis players (Mean ± SD)	Volleyball players (Mean ± SD)	DRIs	P value
Energy (kcal/d)	1930 ± 816	1836 ± 768	1445 ± 693	2139 ± 864	2403	0.23
Protein (g/kg/d)	57 ± 21.3	52 ± 19	53 ± 26	65 ± 22	46	0.22
Thiamine (mg/d)	0.6 ± 0.6	0.5 ± 0.7	0.4 ± 0.5	0.7 ± 0.6	1.1	0.62
Riboflavin (mg/d)	0.7 ± 0.7	0.8 ± 0.9	0.7 ± 0.6	0.6 ± 0.5	1.1	0.76
Niacin (mg/d)	8.7 ± 8.2	8.5 ± 9.1	8.8 ± 11	8.9 ± 6.7	14	0.99
Vitamin B_6 (mg/d)	0.6 ± 0.7	0.6 ± 0.8	0.7 ± 0.9	0.5 ± 0.7	1.3	0.98
VitaminB_{12} (μg/d)	2.0 ± 4.9	2.3 ± 6.8	2.0 ± 3.7	0.3 ± 0.5	2.4	0.36
Folate (μg/d)	82 ± 116	66 ± 61	95 ± 137	96 ± 160	400	0.81
Vitamin C (mg/d)	36 ± 33	43 ± 38	28 ± 18	30 ± 31	75	0.62
Calcium (mg/d)	292 ± 192	360 ± 207	182 ± 124	253 ± 178	1000	0.21
Magnesium (mg/d)	35 ± 23	35 ± 17	48 ± 40	29 ± 21	310	0.38
Iron (mg/d)	7.2 ± 5.8	8.0 ± 7.4	5.8 ± 3.9	6.7 ± 4.3	18	0.77
Zinc (mg/d)	2.2 ± 3.0	2.8 ± 3.4	3.0 ± 4.8	1.2 ± 1.4	8	0.38

TABLE 4: Nutrient intakes of female team players (n = 26). Dietary Reference Intakes [23].

significantly heavier than volleyball players in our study. However, Gaurav et al. [6] did not find significant difference between BMIs of basketball players and the volleyball players.

Further, our study found significant differences in body fat mass of the players in three teams; volleyball players had lower body fat mass than players from other teams. Likewise, basketball players had significantly higher body fat mass as compared to volleyball players [6]. In contrast, Moysi et al. [1] reported that tennis players had lower fat mass and less fat accumulated in the trunk area.

Moreover, the present study established that the %BF in the tennis players was significantly higher (40.9%) than basketball (30.6%) and volleyball players (26.6%). Malousaris *et al.* [14] also reported that %BF for female volleyball players varied between 11.7% and 27.1%.

Muscle mass did not vary among the female players from different teams in our study. According to Ermin [4], there were no signi?cant differences in lean body mass between the female tennis players and non-tennis players. Arabi et al. [1] showed that lean body mass was greater in boys than girls, whereas fat mass was greater in girls than boys.

Volleyball players had the highest fitness score and endurance level. While the fitness score of volleyball players was significantly higher than tennis players, the difference in the endurance level of the three team players was not statistically significant. On the contrary, Byoung and Ju-Hak [3] reported that basketball players have higher endurance level than volleyball players attributing this difference to the practice of the physical activity and endurance training.

The present study showed that the overall energy, vitamins and minerals intakes of most the players were less than the recommended allowances. However, the average intakes of protein and zinc were adequate and marginally exceeded the DRIs. Further, similar nutrient inadequacies existed in the players across different players. The mean energy intake was 1930 kcal/day in contrast to recommended 2139 kcal/day with an energy deficit of almost 200 kcal/day. Hinton et al. [1] reported adequate energy intake in female sports players. The protein intake was 57 g/day in our players in comparison to 87.8 g/day Similarly, the mean intakes of the vitamins and minerals (except zinc) were relatively lower to the intakes of university female sports players in Columbia [10]. Garcin et al. [5] demonstrated a low energy intake, imbalance of protein and fat and insufficient minerals and vitamins in sport players. Marquart et al. [2] also supported the current findings and demonstrated that physically active individuals, as compared with their less active counterparts, fail to consume a diet that contains adequate amounts of vitamins and minerals, which leads to marginal nutrient deficiency and results in substandard training and impaired performance.

5. Conclusion

The differences in body composition were obvious among the players in the three teams. Tennis players had higher BMI, body fat mass and percent body fat; volleyball players had higher fitness score as well as endurance level. The overall intakes of energy and micronutrients among the three teams were less than the recommended allowances and did not differ with the type of sports played.

Due to time constraint, the present study was limited to a sports club in one emirate of UAE, it is recommended that a large-scale study should be designed to include a representative sample at the national level.

6. Acknowledgments

We extend our gratitude to Ms. Khawla Al Serkal, Director of Sharjah Ladies Club for facilitating the execution of our research. Moreover, we extend our appreciation to Ms. Alaa Nawar at Department of Physiotherapy in, University of Sharjah for facilitating the procedures of Modified Canadian Aerobic Fitness Test.

References

[1] A. Arabi, H. Tamim, M. Nabulsi et al., "Sex differences in the effect of body-composition variables on bone mass in healthy children and adolescents.," *American Journal of Clinical Nutrition*, vol. 80, no. 5, pp. 1428–1435, 2004.

[2] D. Brodie, V. Moscrip, and R. Hutcheon, "Body composition measurement: a review of hydrodensitometry, anthropometry, and impedance methods," *Nutrition Journal*, vol. 14, no. 3, pp. 296–310, 1998.

[3] K. Byoung and K. Ju-Hak, "Physical Fitness Profiles of Elite Ball Game Athletes," *International Journal of Applied Sports Sciences*, vol. 17, pp. 71–87, 2005.

[4] K. Ermin, S. Owens, M. A. Ford, and M. Bass, "Bone mineral density of adolescent female tennis players and nontennis players," *Journal of Osteoporosis*, vol. 2012, Article ID 423910, 2012.

[5] M. Garcin, L. Doussot, L. Mille-Hamard, and V. Billat, "Athletes' dietary intake was closer to French RDA's than those of young sedentary counterparts," *Nutrition Research*, vol. 29, no. 10, pp. 736–742, 2009.

[6] V. Gaurav, S. Mandeep, and S. Sukhdev, "Anthropometric characteristics, somatotyping and body composition of volleyball and basketball players," *Journal of Physical Education*, vol. 1, no. 3, pp. 28–32, 2010.

[7] M. N. Hassapidou and A. Manstrantoni, "Dietary intakes of elite female athletes in Greece," *Journal of Human Nutrition and Dietetics*, vol. 14, no. 5, pp. 391–396, 2001.

[8] S. He Kim, P. Hye Young, K. Woo Kyung, and P. Ock Jin, "Nutritional status, iron deficiency related indices, and immunity of female athletes," *Journal of the Academy*

of Nutrition and Dietetics, vol. 18, pp. 86–90, 2002.

[9] H. F. Heather, E. M. Alan, H. F. Heather, and E. M. Alan, *Practical Applications in Sports Nutrition*, vol. 351, 417–428, Jones and Bartlett Learning, MA, 4th edition, 2014.

[10] P. S. Hinton, T. C. Sanford, M. M. Davidson, O. F. Yakushko, and N. C. Beck, "Nutrient intakes and dietary behaviors of male and female collegiate athletes," *International Journal of Sport Nutrition and Exercise Metabolism*, vol. 14, no. 4, pp. 389–405, 2004.

[11] B. Kelly, A. E. Bauman, and L. A. Baur, "Population estimates of Australian children's exposure to food and beverage sponsorship of sports clubs," *Journal of Science and Medicine in Sport*, vol. 17, no. 4, pp. 394–398, 2014.

[12] A. Kuspinar, R. E. Andersen, S. Y. Teng, M. Asano, and N. E. Mayo, "Predicting exercise capacity through submaximal fitness tests in persons with multiple sclerosis," *Archives of Physical Medicine and Rehabilitation*, vol. 91, no. 9, pp. 1410–1417, 2010.

[13] R. D. Lee and D. C. Nieman, *Nutritional assessment*, Mac Graw Hill, 6th edition, 2013.

[14] G. G. Malousaris, N. K. Bergeles, K. G. Barzouka, I. A. Bayios, G. P. Nassis, and M. D. Koskolou, "Somatotype, size and body composition of competitive female volleyball players," *Journal of Science and Medicine in Sport*, vol. 11, no. 3, pp. 337–344, 2008.

[15] J. Sanchis-Moysi, C. Dorado, G. Vicente-Rodríguez, L. Milutinovic, G. L. Garces, and J. A. L. Calbet, "Inter-arm asymmetry in bone mineral content and bone area in postmenopausal recreational tennis players," *Maturitas*, vol. 48, no. 3, pp. 289–298, 2004.

[16] L. Marquart, E. Cohen, and S. Short, "Nutrition knowledge of athletes and their coaches and surveys of dietary intake," *Nutrition in exercise and sport*, vol. 14, pp. 296–310, 1998.

[17] R. U. Newton, W. J. Kraemer, and K. Häkkinen, "Effects of ballistic training on preseason preparation of elite volleyball players," *Medicine & Science in Sports & Exercise*, vol. 31, no. 2, pp. 323–330, 1999.

[18] G. Olivier and M. Gregoirep, "Physical Determinants Of Tennis Performance In Competitive Teenager Players," *Journal of Strength and Conditioning Research*, vol. 23, pp. 1867–1872, 2009.

[19] J. Pařízková, "Body fat and physical fitness," *Nijhoff: The Hague*, pp. 32–37, 1977.

[20] N. T. Rahmawati, S. Budiharjo, and K. Ashizawa, "Somatotypes of young male athletes and non-athlete students in Yogyakarta, Indonesia," *Anthropological Science*, vol. 115, no. 1, pp. 1–7, 2007.

[21] F. E. Thompson and A. F. Subar, *Nutrition in the prevention and treatment of disease*, Academic Press, San Diego, 2nd edition, 2008.

[22] E. Whitney and SR. Rolfes, *Understanding Nutrition. 14e. Canada*, Cengage Learning, 2016.

[23] WHO, Obesity: preventing and managing the global epidemic. Report of a WHO Consultation. WHO Technical Report Series 894. World Health Organization, Geneva. 2000.

3

Weight Management for Athletes: Important Things to be Considered

Chara Odysseos and Maria Avraamidou

Department of Life and Health Sciences, University of Nicosia, Cyprus

Corresponding Author: Maria Avraamidou; email: chara_932@hotmail.com

Abstract

Weight management is difficult for most individuals, as indicated by the high numbers of obesity around the world. Obesity has increased dramatically over the past decades. Unfortunately, this epidemic is not limited to adults but also to children in both globally and Cyprus. Developing a weight management plan is essential for everyone. Regarding to an athlete, weight management is an increasingly integral part, as consuming the right kind of food can lead them in success or failure. The special nutritional needs of athletes are depending on the sport. The most important priority for them is to establish a well-chosen nutrition program based on the type of the sport; the training load and the competitions needs. Health professionals and sport nutritionists need to understand dynamic energy balance and be prepared with effective and evidence-based dietary approaches to help athletes and active individuals achieve their body-weight goals. Therefore, the following review aiming to examine the most recent published data for weight-management both elite and recreational athletes of all ages, and to set out the most appropriate weight-management guidelines and dietary strategies to help them apply this knowledge to the practicalities of their own sport and individual situation.

Keywords: Diet, Athletes, Behavior, Sports

1. Introduction

Weight management is difficult for most individuals, as indicated by the high numbers of obesity around the world [48]. Obesity is a global health epidemic characterized by excessive body fat accumulation [20]. Individuals with body mass index (BMI) falling within 25-29.9kg/m^{2}are indicated as overweight, whereas individuals with BMI at or above 30kg/m^2 are indicated as obese [41]. Based on a study conducted in 2014, revealed that within four decades the global obesity in men has tripled, from 3.2% in 1975 to 10.8% in 2014 [43]. During the same period, obesity in women has more than doubled from 6.4% in 1975 to 14.9% in 2014.

Unfortunately, the obesity epidemic is not limited to adults. Currently, 32 % of children between the ages of 2 and 19 years are above the 85 % percentile for BMI for age [29]. Published data have documented that there is severe obesity problem in children in Cyprus over the past decade, making childhood obesity one of the most crucial public health problems in our country [41]. In a recent study conducted in 2010, 20.1% of Cypriot children between the ages of 6-12 were found obese, up from 16.5% in 2000. Similarly, obesity rates within the same group raised from 5.9% in 2000, to 8.1% in 2010 which means that more young athletes will come to their sport fatter than considered desirable for optimal performance [41].

Developing a weight management plan is essential for everyone. Proper nutrition plays an important role at peak performance, specifically when someone does exercise to keep fit, participate regularly in organized sports activities or training to reach the top level of the sport. With regard to an athlete, weight management is an increasingly integral part, as consuming the right kind of food can lead individually in the success or failure [52]. If athletes combine serious restriction energy with a strong resistance and strength training program, then it can actually lead to metabolic changes. These two factors are extremely stressful for the athletes due to lose rapid body weight, also minimized their sports performance, and dangerous about their health [23].

The special nutritional needs of athletes are depending on the sport; whether they want to lose body fat or gaining and/or maintaining lean tissue [23]. While some athletes appear to be naturally lean, with weight and body size well matched for their sport, others need to change their weight and/or body composition to be competitive. For instance, aesthetic sports e.g. rhythmic and artistic gymnastics, ice-skating or dancing, weight division sports e.g. judo, or rowing gym sports e.g. aerobics, endurance sports e.g. long distance running are sports requiring low body-weight and/or body composition in order to considered an athlete as elite [56].

The most important priority for athletes is to establish a well-chosen nutrition program based on the type of the sport, body composition goals about the sport, also the training load and the competition needs [5]. A proper athletic diet will provide adequate nutrients and energy to enhance adaptations from training, support optimal recovery with no food-related stress. It is known that heavy training, requires more nutrients and energy mainly in carbohydrate, protein and micronutrients (vitamins and minerals) [5].

Health professionals and sport nutritionists need to understand dynamic energy balance and be prepared with effective and evidence-based dietary approaches to help athletes and active individuals achieve their body-weight goals [23]. Therefore, the aim of this review is to examine the most recent published articles for weight-management both elite and recreational athletes of all ages, and also to set out the most appropriate weight-management guidelines to help them apply this knowledge to the practicalities of their own sport and individual situation.

2. Weight – Control Behavior in Athletes

In general, most athletes who want to lose weight fall into two categories; those who are overweight or obese based on body-fat levels, and those who are already lean, but desire additional body fat loss. Some of these athletes fall into weight-sensitive (e.g., endurance athletes, ski jumping), weight-class (e.g., wrestling, judo), or aesthetically judged (e.g., gymnastics, figure skating) sports [46].

It is known that excess body fat decreasing athletic performance as well as could increase the risk of chronic diseases for athletes. One study found that 21% of first Division college football players were obese and had insulin resistance, while 9% had metabolic syndrome. Thus, for these athletes, weight loss could improve performance and prevent the development of serious chronic diseases [3].

Conversely, many elite and recreational athletes who have normal weight or low body weights, yet they still want to lose weight in order to improve their performance and/or to achieve a body shape for aesthetic reasons [46]. Some of these individuals are young and still growing, which is the least desirable time to severely restrict energy intake while participating in high levels of exercise [24].

Restrict weight control and diet low in calories are particularly widespread in sports where focus in leanness (leanness-sports) or low body weight like aesthetic or endurance sports . One study showed that NCAA Division I athletes who competing in leanness sports, had significantly higher on the sub-score for Body Dissatisfaction and had lower mean desired body weight than those competing in non-leanness sports [35]. This study was in line with Rosendahl et al. [39] who compare leanness sports and non-leanness sports concluded that athletes competing in leanness sports scored higher for weight-control behaviour than those competing in non-leanness sports.

On the other hand, a study with 204 NCAA Division I, athletes of many sports types using the Questionnaire for Eating Disorder Diagnosis showed that over half of the athletes were not satisfied with their body weight. More of them wanted to lose weight (~5.9 kg), and also there was a weight fluctuation of more than 10% within a year of the athletes. They stated that the methods they used to reduce their body weight were exercise around 2 hours a day and the fasting or on a low calories diet [16].

Martinsen et al. [24] had 606 elite athletes from 50 different sports types who showed similar frequencies of pathogenic weight-control methods like vomiting, laxatives, diuretics and diet pills. It seemed that between female and male athletes, the female athletes used more these pathogenic weight-control methods. When looking at weight concerns, the 24% of the female athletes and 7.5% of the male athletes were presently on a diet and have been on a diet at least three times before due to this reason.

In addition, for athletes in aesthetic sports like figure skaters, synchronized swimmers, gymnasts, maintaining a low body weight over a competitive season without injury or illness or the use of extreme weight-control methods is also a challenge [45]. In a study of psychosocial correlates of bulimic symptoms were participated 280 NCAA Division I female gymnasts and 134 NCAA Division I female swimmers/divers showed that the level of body dissatisfaction, as well as restrictive eating, was related to the amount of experienced pressure from teammates and coaches [1].

Other study showed that there was no difference about the weight-concerns between the synchronized swimmers and other "non-weight dependent sports types" such as basketball, volleyball, soccer [13].

However, it seemed that it can be difficult to manage safe weight loss in athletes who need to meet a designated weight on competition day, like lightweight rowers, jockeys, or wrestlers. These individuals typically weight cycle, with their weight fluctuating dramatically between the competitive and off seasons [58], (Berkovich et al. 2016).

Looking at weight-dependent sports, three studies described methods of rapid weight-control amongst judo athletes and one study for Taekwondo. The first one where was among elite male and female judo athletes showed that 86% have reduced body weight rapidly before the competition (around 2-5%), with some athletes losing up to 10% ten times or more in their careers [2]. The fluctuation of weight was confirmed with a study of Rouveix et al. [40] which showed that quick weight reduction is an inherent part of the judo athletes. Also, 70% of the athletes seemed that lost more than 2.8 kg during a season, with the methods of excessive exercises or limit the food and fluids consumption.

Moreover, in a cross-sectional study of Berkovich et al. (2016) were used 108 male athletes from local judo teams. Rapid Weight Loss (RWL) was practiced by 80% of the athletes before competition, beginning at an average age of 12.5 ± 2.2 years with the highest prevalence (~94%) in the oldest group of judoka (16–17.9 years). Pre-competition weight loss duration was 8 ± 5.4 days, with an average weight reduction of 1.5 ± 1.1 kg. The number of weight loss efforts per athlete in the past season was

2.8 ± 2.2. RWL was achieved by increased physical activity (82.6%), skipped meals (56.3%), or fasting at least once (47%). Two-thirds of the athletes indicated that they experienced pressure from their coaches and were the most influential figure in their decision to lose weight before competition. These athletes used the methods which compromised nutritional status, diminished physical performance and impaired growth and development. These methods can potentially lead to significant health risks. A key priority for the persons who guide young adults in weight loss for competitive sports is to have the knowledge and understanding to make safe recommendations and appropriate decisions about achieving specific and healthy weight goals.

Moreover, Sandos et al. (2016) investigated the prevalence, magnitude, and methods of quick weight loss among 72 male and 44 female Taekwondo athletes from all competitive levels. The results from the given questionnaires have shown that among the male athletes, 77.4% of the regional/state level and 75.6% of the national/international athletes declared to have reduced weight to compete in lighter weight categories. Among women, 88.9% of regional/state level and 88.6% of national/international level were using rapid weight loss strategies. Athletes reported to usually lose around 3% of their body weight, with some athletes reaching around 7% of their body weight. The methods used to achieve weight loss are potentially dangerous for health and had no difference between sexes. Four methods were more frequently used by men athletes in higher competitive levels as compared to lower levels, as follows: skipping meals, fasting, restricting fluids and spitting. Taekwondo athletes lost around 3% of their body mass, using the health-dangerous methods. Although no difference was found between sexes, while lower level athletes typically skip meals, fast, restrict fluids and spitting. Considering that these health-threating methods are more commonly used by lower level athletes, specific education programs should be directed to them [49].

Another study investigated the methods adopted to reduce body mass (BM) in competitive athletes from the grappling (judo, jujitsu) and striking (karate and taekwondo) combat sports in Brazil. A standardized questionnaire was used with objective questions self-administered to 580 athletes. Regardless of the sport, 60% of the athletes reported using a method of RWL via increased energy expenditure. Strikers tend to begin reducing BM during adolescence. Furthermore, 50% of the sample used saunas and plastic clothing, and only 26.1% received advice from a nutritionist. In addition, a high percentage of athletes use unapproved or prohibited methods such as diuretics, saunas, and plastic clothing [4]. Few athletes are naturally light weight enough for these types of competitive sports, thus weight loss will be required the weeks or days prior to competition [44].

3. Achieving a Healthy and Competitive Body Weight

According to a research conducted in 2015, depending on the sport, the weight of an athlete during the competitive season is usually lower than the weight in off season. As a result of this, most of the athletes restricting their energy intake in order to achieve their competitive weight and they often gain the lost-weight back during the off season [23]. The ultimate goal for everyone and for athletes as well, is to develop healthy eating habits so as to achieve a healthy body weight that they can maintain for most of the year. In that way, athletes reducing the amount of weight that need to be lost for competition. The same research supported that for some sports, losing high amount of weight - for the needs of the competitive season - is not healthy for most athletes. Moreover, Manore [23] continued by saying that the key priority for each athlete is to make sure that their goal-weight is realistic and will not cause any health issues and/or increase the risk of injuries. Taking into consideration their ages as well as the level of their physical development are some ways that can help the athlete identify whether the weight they are trying to achieve is realistic. Sport dietitians are the health professionals should monitor athletes to help them reach their body-weight goals and to assure they are maintaining healthy eating habits [23].

While thinking of dietary strategies, expect to be analyzed evidence-based diet and lifestyle guidelines for athletes who are having a weight-specific goal; whether they are interested in losing weight, maintaining lean tissue and/or preventing weight regain [23]. To be more specific, dietary strategies section will provide to athletes an in-depth to diet and exercise specific behavior changes so as to produce the desired body-weight and composition modifications

4. Energy Restriction Approaches

The approach for restricting energy intake combined with an intense endurance and strength-training program can actually increase metabolic adaptations that slow weight loss and diminish the additive effects of these two factors on weight loss. But, this approach should be avoided because athletes are leading in a number of other negative performance and health consequences [28]. For example, decreased athletic performance effects due to decreased muscle strength, glycogen stores, concentration, coordination and training responses, and increased irritability. Also, increased negative health consequences (injury due to fatigue, loss of lean tissue, poor nutrient intakes, etc), increased risk of disordered eating behaviors, dehydration, and emotional distress due to hunger, fatigue, and stress [15].

It is important to remember that with negative energy balance, lean, fit individuals can quickly lose lean tissue if energy is restricted too dramatically [50]. For instance, one study placed active military personnel (BMI 25 ± 1 kg/m2) on a 40 % energy-restricted diet for 30 days, while being fed the recommended dietary allowance (RDA) for protein (0.8 g/kg/body weight) [30]. Of the 3.3 kg lost during this time (4.2 % body weight), 58 % was lean tissue (1.9 kg). In contrast, when they placed sedentary overweight individuals (BMI 27.8 kg/m2) on a 25 % energy-restriction diet for 3 months, they lost 6 kg, with only 33 % coming from lean tissue (2 kg) [30]. Furthermore, Garthe et al. [15] showed that the athletes who had slower, and more logical weight loss around 0.7 % loss of body weight per week helped maintain lean tissue while improving strength gains compared with more severe weight loss (1.4 % weight loss/week).

Therefore, for the athletes who already have a training, it is preferable to moderately restrict energy intake (e.g., 500–700 kcal/day) and take longer to reach the weight loss goal (0.50-1 kg /week). This approach also allows the time required to adapt to new dietary habits while making sure adequate energy is available for exercise training [15].

5. Timing of food Consumption during Training and throughout the Day

Timing of food intake around exercise training and spreading food intake throughout the day is a key priority for the athlete. This approach ensures that the body has the nutrients and energy needed for the specific exercise and the building and repairing of lean tissue [46]. Furthermore, may delay hunger and as an extension of this may prevent the athlete from consuming foods or beverages not included in their diet plan. It is evidence-based that when athletes are concerned about their weight -particularly female athletes- they usually skipping meals, mainly breakfast [12]. Recent study of Erdman [12] reported that 98% of elite Canadian male athletes consumed breakfast, while Shriver et al. [42] at the same year found that only 23% of elite college female athletes consumed breakfast. The majority of the athletes in the second study reported their diets to be poor, most of the calories were consuming at dinner and they found it difficult to maintain their weight. Those eating habits may be a result of the idea that skipping breakfast will help in reducing caloric intake, therefore the overall weight [42].

Focusing on the athlete, breakfast constitutes the most important meal of the day, mainly due to the fact that it can provide carbohydrates needed to help replenish lost glycogen after an overnight fast and provide the appropriate fuel for exercise [8]. For those who participate in an early-morning workout, eating a light pre-workout snack and a nutritious post-workout breakfast will assure the adequate nutrients have been lost during exercise particularly carbohydrate and protein. In a research examined the importance of breakfast for athletes, it was found that during moderate training weeks, breakfast provided 21% of the daily carbohydrate intake for junior elite triathletes, while during high intensity training weeks, breakfast provided 28% of their daily carbohydrate intake. Therefore, skipping breakfast would lower total daily carbohydrate intake, thus affecting exercise performance [8].

As mentioned above, post-workout meal is crucial as well, since it provides to the athlete all the necessary nutrients for the replenishment of lost glycogen, and also building and repairing their lean tissue. An appropriate post-workout meal should compose of foods high in fluids for rehydration and carbohydrates in the form of low energy dense foods, such as whole fruits and vegetables and whole grains. Sport dietitians should monitor athletes so as to ensure they develop healthy eating habits and prepare the most appropriate diet plan according to the individual needs. Overall, the use of low energy dense diet plan is the most effective way for refueling during training periods, while during competitive periods there is a need for higher energy dense foods if glycogen replacement needs to occur in less than 24 hours [23].

6. Diet Plan for Weight Loss

The possibilities of whether a low in energy dense diet plan is more effective on weight loss for athletes compared with a high energy dense diet plan were examined below.

Generally, this type of diet is lower in fat and reduces or eliminates energy dense beverages particularly sweetened beverages and alcohol [28]. More specifically, a low-energy dense diet is composed with a high consumption of vegetables, whole fruits and grains as well as incorporates low-fat dairy products. This low-fat, high-fiber, high-water diet means an individual still feel satiated even when the overall energy intake is lower, mostly due to the greater volume of food [28]. As reported by many references, when examined the effectiveness of a low-energy diet plan on the overall weight-changes, is expected to observe an overall weight and energy intake reduction, weight regain prevention as well as satiety maintenance [10, 38].

In a follow-up study, Rolls and his colleagues observed the effect of changing portion size, energy density or a combination of the two, on total energy intake over two days [37]. They altered energy density by substituting full fat foods with low fat foods (e.g. whole milk with skim milk) and by changing portions of vegetables. The study concluded that energy density and portion size independently altered energy intake. Reducing portion size by 25%, decreased energy intake by 231kcal / day (10% decreases). Similarly, when energy density was reduced by 25%, energy intake decreased by 575 kcal / day (24% decreases). Therefore, minimizing both energy density and portion size will have the most positive impact on energy intake reduction by 32% [37]. Another similar study has shown this weight loss approach also works in longer dietary interventions. Ledikwe et al. [21] examined 35 obese women consuming a low energy dense diet for one year and 36 obese women consuming low fat diet only for the same period. They found that the first group has lost 20% more weight than the second group. Dietary fat intake was similarly decreased in both groups, but those in the low energy dense group, reported significantly lower ratings of hunger. Physical activity was the same between the groups. Currently, there is no published research reporting the effectiveness of the low energy dense diet for weight loss in athletes. However, only two resent researchers suggest that for highly active females, this diet plan does not provide enough energy to cover the exercise cost and reproductive function [18, 34]. The satiating effect of these diets combined with the hunger effects of intense exercise may contribute to the energy deficiency of this group of athletes.

Overall, lowering the energy dense of the diet is preferable at reducing energy intake rather than lowering portion size. For athletes following a lower energy dense diet could help them maintain their weight loss. A key component of a low energy dense eating plan is to promote satiation by increasing the intake of foods high in water and fiber, while reducing the intake of high fat foods [18].

7. Consumption of Energy Dense Beverages

Consumption of energy dense beverages and alcohol increase the overall daily energy in a diet plan, but it has been shown that there is a reduction in satiety and incomplete energy compensation [18]. Removing those beverages from the diet may help athletes achieve their weight-goals without making any other dietary changes. For these athletes, sweetened beverages (e.g., sport drinks) should be limited to meet the recommended consumption for hydration and fueling when participating in sport [18].

8. Protein Intake, Quality, and Timing

When the energy intake is restricted, it is easy for protein intake to decrease while protein needs to increase with energy restriction in order to help the preservation of skeletal muscle integrity, especially as regards physically active individuals [7].

Generally, athletes have increased protein needs compared with non-active individuals (1.4–1.7 g/protein/kg and 0.8 g/protein/kg respectively) [19, 36]. The volume and type of exercise as well as the level of energy restriction will determine the amount of additional protein needed [7] . For example, Mettler et al. [26] demonstrated that increasing dietary protein during periods of severe energy restriction can help in the maintenance of lean tissue in active individuals participating in strength training during dieting. For 1 week, they placed 20 healthy resistance-trained male athletes on an energy-restricted diet (60 % of habitual energy intake). During this time, they were randomly assigned to two groups, either in the control group (1 g/protein/kg; $n = 10$) or in the treatment group (2.3 g/protein/kg; $n = 10$). The results derived from the above study showed that the loss of lean mass was greater in the control group (−1.6 kg in 1 week) than in the treatment group (−0.3 kg). Thus, the higher protein intake (~35 % of energy intake) helped preserve lean tissue when energy intake was severely restricted for a short time.

In addition, athletes need to consume adequate high-quality protein throughout the day, but especially after exercise and at breakfast [57]. Spreading protein intake throughout the day is beneficial for weight loss for athlete by ensuring that adequate protein amount is constantly available for building, repair, and maintenance of lean tissue. In addition, higher protein diets have been associated with increased satiety and reductions in energy intake. Weigle et al. [55] reported a decrease in energy intake (−441 ± 64 kcal/day) over a 12-week period in healthy sedentary individuals fed an ad libitum high-protein diet (30 % energy from protein, 20 % fat, and 50 % carbohydrate) compared with an isocaloric lower protein diet (15 % of energy from protein). Although, most athletes consume high amounts of protein, they may not get this protein after exercise and spread it out throughout the day. It may be more usual for the majority of the energy and protein to be consumed in a large meal at the end of the day [22].

9. Conclusions

Taking all into consideration, weight management for athletes can be difficult, and in sometimes risky for the health. Despite the fact that they spend high amounts of energy in the training, they may still need to monitor diet and lifestyle to maintain a competitive body weight. If an athlete needs to lose weight, working with a supportive health care team such as coach, sports medicine team, and sport dietitian will help ensure success. Furthermore, a registered dietitian trained in sports nutrition should be collaborate with the coaches in order to help the athlete identify and reach a realistic goal weight with making an individualized daily meal plans, address nutrition and sport supplements and health issues, and make sure the athletes is fueled appropriately for their sport. To provide a consistent message to the athlete, all health professionals need to understand the many physiological and environmental factors influencing body weight and energy balance. This will improve their ability to design personalized and realistic weight-management programs.

References

[1] C. M. Anderson, T. A. Petrie, and C. S. Neumann, "Psychosocial correlates of bulimic symptoms among NCAA division-I female collegiate gymnasts and swimmers/divers," *Journal of Sport & Exercise Psychology* , vol. 33, no. 4, pp. 483–505, 2011.

[2] G. Giannini Artioli, B. Gualano, E. Franchini et al., "Prevalence, magnitude, and methods of rapid weight loss among judo competitors," *Medicine & Science in Sports & Exercise*, vol. 42, no. 3, pp. 436–442, 2010.

[3] J. R. Borchers, K. L. Clem, D. L. Habash, H. N. Nagaraja, L. M. Stokley, and T. M. Best, "Metabolic syndrome and insulin resistance in division 1 collegiate football players," *Medicine & Science in Sports & Exercise*, vol. 41, no. 12, pp. 2105–2110, 2009.

[4] C. J. Brito, A. F. C. M. Roas, I. S. S. Brito, J. C. B. Marins, C. Córdova, and E. Franchini, "Methods of body-mass reduction by combat sport athletes," *International Journal of Sport Nutrition and Exercise Metabolism*, vol. 22, no. 2, pp. 89–97, 2012.

[5] L. M. Burke, G. R. Cox, N. K. Cummings, and B. Desbrow, "Guidelines for daily carbohydrate intake: Do athletes achieve them?" *Sports Medicine*, vol. 31, no. 4, pp. 267–299, 2001.

[6] Canadian Sport Institute Ontario (2015), Sport Nutritionist. Retrieves 17 December 2016, from http://www.csipacific.ca/wp-content/uploads/201508CSIOSportNutritionistMatCover.pdf.

[7] J. W. Carbone, J. P. McClung, and S. M. Pasiakos, "Skeletal muscle responses to negative energy balance: Effects of dietary protein," *Advances in Nutrition*, vol. 3, no. 2, pp. 119–126, 2012.

[8] A. Carlsohn, S. Nippe, J. Heydenreich, and F. Mayer, "Carbohydrate intake and food sources of junior triathletes during a moderate and an intensive training period," *International Journal of Sport Nutrition and Exercise Metabolism*, vol. 22, no. 6, pp. 438–443, 2012.

[9] J. E. Donnelly, S. N. Blair, J. M. Jakicic, M. M. Manore, J. W. Rankin, and B. K. Smith, "Appropriate physical activity intervention strategies for weight loss and prevention of weight regain for adults," *Medicine & Science in Sports & Exercise*, vol. 41, no. 2, pp. 459–471, 2009.

[10] J. A. Ello-Martin, J. H. Ledikwe, and B. J. Rolls, "The influence of food portion size and energy density on energy intake: implications for weight management.," *American Journal of Clinical Nutrition*, vol. 82, no. 1, 2005.

[11] J. A. Ello-Martin, L. S. Roe, J. H. Ledikwe et al., "Dietary energy density in the treatment of obesity: a year-long trial comparing 2 weight-loss diets," *Am J Clin Nutr*, vol. 85, pp. 1465–1477, 2007.

[12] K. A. Erdman, J. Tunnicliffe, V. M. Lun, and R. A. Reimer, "Eating patterns and composition of meals and snacks in elite Canadian athletes," *International Journal of Sport Nutrition and Exercise Metabolism*, vol. 23, no. 3, pp. 210–219, 2013.

[13] C. Ferrand, C. Magnan, and R. A. Philippe, "Body-esteem, body mass index, and risk for disordered eating among adolescents in synchronized swimming," *Perceptual and Motor Skills*, vol. 101, no. 3, pp. 877–884, 2005.

[14] E. Franchini, C. J. Brito, and G. G. Artioli, "Weight loss in combat sports: Physiological, psychological and performance effects," *Journal of the International Society of Sports Nutrition*, vol. 9, article no. 52, 2012.

[15] I. Garthe, T. Raastad, P. E. Refsnes, A. Koivisto, and J. Sundgot-Borgen, "Effect of two different weight-loss rates on body composition and strength and power-related performance in elite athletes," *International Journal of Sport Nutrition and Exercise Metabolism*, vol. 21, no. 2, pp. 97–104, 2011.

[16] C. Greenleaf, T. Petrie, J. Carter, and J. Reel, "Female collegiate athletes: Prevalence of eating disorders and disordered eating behaviors," *Journal of American College Health*, vol. 57, no. 5, pp. 489–495, 2009.

[17] E. R. Helms, C. Zinn, D. S. Rowlands, and S. R. Brown, "A systematic review of dietary protein during caloric restriction in resistance trained lean athletes: A case for higher intakes," *International Journal of Sport Nutrition and Exercise Metabolism*, vol. 24, no. 2, pp. 127–138, 2014.

[18] S. M. Howe, T. M. Hand, and M. M. Manore, "Exercise-trained men and women: Role of exercise and diet on appetite and energy intake," *Nutrients*, vol. 6, no. 11, pp. 4935–4960, 2014.

[19] Institute of Medicine (IOM) Food and Nutrition Board, *Dietary Reference Intakes for Energy, Carbohydrate, Fiber, Fat, Fatty Acids, Cholesterol, Protein, and Amino Acids (Macronutrients)*, National Academies Press, Washington, D.C., 2005.

[20] I. Kyriazis, M. Rekleiti, M. Saridi et al., "Prevalence of obesity in children aged 6-12 years in Greece: Nutritional behaviour and physical activity," *Archives of Medical Science*, vol. 8, no. 5, pp. 859–864, 2012.

[21] J. A. Ello-Martin, J. H. Ledikwe, and B. J. Rolls, "The influence of food portion size and energy density on energy intake: implications for weight management," *American Journal of Clinical Nutrition*, vol. 82, no. 1, 2005.

[22] M. M. Manore, N. L. Meyer, and J. Thompson, *Sport nutrition for health and performance*, Human Kinetics, Champaign, 2nd edition, 2009.

[23] M. M. Manore, "Weight Management for Athletes and Active Individuals: A Brief Review," *Sports Medicine*, vol. 45, pp. 83–92, 2015.

[24] M. Martinsen, S. Bratland-Sanda, A. K. Eriksson, and J. Sundgot-Borgen, "Dieting to win or to be thin? A study of dieting and disordered eating among adolescent elite athletes and non-athlete controls," *British Journal of Sports Medicine*, vol. 44, no. 1, pp. 70–76, 2010.

[25] S. H. Mendes, A. C. Tritto, J. P. L. P. Guilherme et al., "Effect of rapid weight loss on performance in combat sport male athletes: does adaptation to chronic weight cycling play a role?" *British Journal of Sports Medicine*, vol. 47, no. 18, pp. 1155–1160, 2013.

[26] S. Mettler, N. Mitchell, and K. D. Tipton, "Increased protein intake reduces lean body mass loss during weight loss in athletes," *Medicine & Science in Sports & Exercise*, vol. 42, no. 2, pp. 326–337, 2010.

[27] M. Khodaee, L. Olewinski, B. Shadgan, and R. R. Kiningham, "Rapid weight loss in sports with weight classes," *Current Sports Medicine Reports*, vol. 14, no. 6, pp. 435–441, 2015.

[28] M. Mountjoy, J. Sundgot-Borgen, L. Burke et al., "The IOC consensus statement: Beyond the Female Athlete Triad-Relative Energy Deficiency in Sport (RED-S)," *British Journal of Sports Medicine*, vol. 48, no. 7, pp. 491–497, 2014.

[29] C. L. Ogden, M. D. Carroll, L. R. Curtin, M. M. Lamb, and K. M. Flegal, "Prevalence of high body mass index in US children and adolescents, 2007-2008," *The Journal of the American Medical Association*, vol. 303, no. 3, pp. 242–249, 2010.

[30] S. M. Pasiakos, J. J. Cao, L. M. Margolis et al., "Effects of high-protein diets on fat-free mass and muscle protein synthesis following weight loss: A randomized controlled trial," *The FASEB Journal*, vol. 27, no. 9, pp. 3837–3847, 2013.

[31] S. Pettersson, M. Pipping Ekström, and C. M. Berg, "The food and weight combat. A problematic fight for the elite combat sports athlete," *Appetite*, vol. 59, no. 2, pp. 234–242, 2012.

[32] R. Reale, G. Slater, and L. M. Burke, "Acute Weight Loss Strategies for Combat Sports and Applications to Olympic Success," *Human Kinetics*, pp. 30–10, 2016.

[33] L. M. Redman, L. K. Heilbronn, C. K. Martin et al., "Metabolic and behavioral compensations in response to caloric restriction: implications for the maintenance of weight loss," *PLoS ONE*, vol. 4, no. 2, Article ID e4377, 2009.

[34] J. L. Reed, J. L. Bowell, B. R. Hill, B. A. Williams, M. J. de Souza, and N. I. Williams, "Exercising women with menstrual disturbances consume low energy dense foods and beverages," *Applied Physiology, Nutrition, and Metabolism*, vol. 36, no. 3, pp. 382–394, 2011.

[35] M. F. Reinking and L. E. Alexander, "Prevalence of disordered-eating behaviors in undergraduate female collegiate athletes and nonathletes," *Journal of Athletic Training*, vol. 40, no. 1, pp. 47–51, 2005.

[36] N. R. Rodriguez, N. M. DiMarco, and S. Langley, "Position of the American dietetic association, dietitians of Canada, and the american college of sports medicine: nutrition and athletic performance," *Journal of the Academy of Nutrition and Dietetics*, vol. 109, no. 3, pp. 509–527, 2009.

[37] BJ. Rolls, LS. Roe, and JS. Meengs, "Reductions in portion size and energy density of foods are additive and lead to sustained decreases in energy intake," *Am J Clin Nutr*, vol. 83, pp. 11–17, 2006.

[38] B. J. Rolls, "The relationship between dietary energy density and energy intake," *Physiology & Behavior*, vol. 97, no. 5, pp. 609–615, 2009.

[39] J. Rosendahl, B. Bormann, K. Aschenbrenner, F. Aschenbrenner, and B. Strauss, "Dieting and disordered eating in German high school athletes and non-athletes," *Scandinavian Journal of Medicine & Science in Sports*, vol. 19, no. 5, pp. 731–739, 2009.

[40] M. Rouveix, M. Bouget, C. Pannafieux, S. Champely, and E. Filaire, "Eating attitudes, body esteem, perfectionism and anxiety of judo athletes and nonathletes," *International Journal of Sports Medicine*, vol. 28, no. 4, pp. 340–345, 2007.

[41] C. Savva, YA. Kourides, and C. Hadjigeorgiou, "Overweight and obesity prevalence and trends in children and adolescents in Cyprus 2000-201," *Obesity Research & Clinical Prcactice*, vol. 8, pp. 426–434, 2013.

[42] L. H. Shriver, N. M. Betts, and G. Wollenberg, "Dietary intakes and eating habits of college athletes: Are female college athletes following the current sports nutrition standards?" *Journal of American College Health*, vol. 61, no. 1, pp. 10–16, 2013.

[43] G. M. Singh, G. Danaei, F. Farzadfar et al., "The Age-Specific Quantitative Effects of Metabolic Risk Factors on Cardiovascular Diseases and Diabetes: A Pooled Analysis," *PLoS ONE*, vol. 8, no. 7, p. e65174, 2013.

[44] G. J. Slater, A. J. Rice, K. Sharpe, I. Mujika, D. Jenkins, and A. G. Hahn, "Body-mass management of Australian lightweight rowers prior to and during competition," *Medicine & Science in Sports & Exercise*, vol. 37, no. 5, pp. 860–866, 2005.

[45] J. Sundgot-Borgen and I. Garthe, "Elite athletes in aesthetic and Olympic weight-class sports and the challenge of body weight and body composition," *Journal of Sports Sciences*, vol. 29, no. 1, pp. S101–S114, 2011.

[46] J. Sundgot-Borgen, N. L. Meyer, T. G. Lohman et al., "How to minimise the health risks to athletes who compete in weight-sensitive sports review and position statement on behalf of the Ad Hoc Research Working Group on Body Composition, Health and Performance, under the auspices of the IOC Medical Commission," *British Journal of Sports Medicine*, vol. 47, no. 16, pp. 1012–1022, 2013.

[47] J. Sundgot-Borgen and M. K. Torstveit, "Aspects of disordered eating continuum in elite high-intensity sports," *Scandinavian Journal of Medicine & Science in Sports*, vol. 20, no. 2, pp. 112–121, 2010.

[48] B. A. Swinburn, G. Sacks, K. D. Hall et al., "The global obesity pandemic: shaped by global drivers and local environments," *The Lancet*, vol. 378, no. 9793, pp. 804–814, 2011.

[49] J. F. Silva Santos, M. Y. Takito, G. G. Artioli, and E. Franchini, "Weight loss practices in Taekwondo athletes of different competitive levels," *Journal of Exercise Rehabilitation*, vol. 12, no. 3, pp. 202–208, 2016.

[50] D. Thomas, S. Das, J. A. Levine et al., "New fat free mass - fat mass model for use in physiological energy balance equations," *Nutrition & Metabolism*, vol. 7, no. 1, p. 39, 2010.

[51] K. D. Tipton and L. J. C. van Loon, "Nutritional Coaching Strategy to Modulate Training Efficiency," in *75th Nestlé Nutrition Institute Workshop*, pp. 123–133, Mallorca, 2013.

[52] K. D. Tipton and R. R. Wolfe, "Protein and amino acids for athletes," *Journal of Sports Sciences*, vol. 22, no. 1, pp. 65–79, 2004.

[53] E. T. Trexler, A. E. Smith-Ryan, and L. E. Norton, "Metabolic adaptation to weight loss: implications for the athlete," *J Int Soc Sports Nutr*, p. 11, 2013.

[54] P. S. Turocy, B. F. DePalma, C. A. Horswill et al., "National athletic trainers' association position statement: Safe weight loss and maintenance practices in sport and exercise," *Journal of Athletic Training*, vol. 46, no. 3, pp. 322–336, 2011.

[55] D. S. Weigle, P. A. Breen, C. C. Matthys et al., "A high-protein diet induces sustained reductions in appetite, ad libitum caloric intake, and body weight despite compensatory changes in diurnal plasma leptin and ghrelin concentrations," *American Journal of Clinical Nutrition*, vol. 82, no. 1, pp. 41–48, 2005.

[56] A. Werner, A. Thiel, S. Schneider, J. Mayer, K. E. Giel, and S. Zipfel, "Weight-control behaviour and weight-concerns in young elite athletes - a systematic review," *Journal of Eating Disorders*, vol. 1, no. 1, article no. 18, 2013.

[57] M. S. Westerterp-Plantenga, A. Nieuwenhuizen, D. Tomé, S. Soenen, and K. R. Westerterp, "Dietary protein, weight loss, and weight maintenance," *Annual Review of Nutrition*, vol. 29, no. 1, pp. 21–41, 2009.

[58] G. Wilson, B. Drust, J. P. Morton, and G. L. Close, "Weight-making strategies in professional jockeys: Implications for physical and mental health and well-being," *Sports Medicine*, vol. 44, no. 6, pp. 785–796, 2014.

[59] L. Woodroffe, J. J. Donnenwerth, and A. R. Peterson, "Weight Management Counseling for Wrestling Athletes," in *Pediatr Ann*, vol. 45, no. 3, pp. e87–e90, 2016.

4

The Role of Genetic, Dietary and Lifestyle Factors in Pediatric Metabolic Syndrome: A Review of the Literature from Prenatal to Adolescence

Teresa Arora[1,2], Sahar Agouba[2], Ahmad Sharara[2], and Shahrad Taheri[2]

[1]Zayed University, Department of Psychology, Abu Dhabi, United Arab Emirates
[2]Weill Cornell Medicine in Qatar, Clinical Research Core, Doha, Qatar

Corresponding Author: Teresa Arora; email: Teresa.Arora@zu.ac.ae

Abstract

The metabolic syndrome (MetS) is described as a cluster of health conditions that are associated with an increased risk of cardiovascular disease. The clinical diagnosis of MetS in pediatrics is challenging due to differing criteria, although the estimated prevalence continues to rise. The increased prevalence of childhood obesity and insulin resistance, in both developed and developing countries, is believed to be a major contributor to MetS diagnosis in children. We review the current literature surrounding genetic predisposition, maternal influence, epigenetics, environmental and lifestyle factors pertaining to pediatric MetS with a specific emphasis on obesity and insulin resistance. We highlight and discuss recent, key studies in prenatal through to adolescent populations and review evidence suggesting that children may be pre-disposed to obesity and insulin resistance, prenatally. We also discuss several key lifestyle drivers of these conditions including poor nutrition and dietary habits, insufficient physical activity, use of electronic devices, over-consumption of caffeinated and/or sugar-sweetened beverages, as well as the importance of sleep during childhood and adolescence in relation to metabolic health. We conclude with recommendations for preventable methods to tackle this growing pediatric public health issue, which, if current trends continue, will undoubtedly compromise the health and longevity of the next adult generation.

Keywords: metabolic syndrome, obesity, pediatrics, diet, physical activity

1. Introduction

The metabolic syndrome is a constellation of cardio-metabolic abnormalities that were observed to cluster and increase cardiovascular risk. Several hypotheses have been proposed suggesting common etiological mechanisms for the metabolic syndrome revolving around central adiposity and insulin resistance. The components of the metabolic syndrome depend on the definitions used by various international bodies. Generally, components include: 1) elevated triglycerides; 2) low levels of high density lipoprotein-cholesterol (HDL-C); 3) hypertension; 4) glucose intolerance/insulin resistance; and 5) excess adiposity (usually determined through waist circumference or body mass index (BMI) cut points). If an individual has three or more components, they are designated to have the metabolic syndrome.

The metabolic syndrome is usually observed in older populations, but with an increasing prevalence of obesity in younger populations, it is becoming more common in younger individuals with potentially serious downstream repercussions for health. The definition of the metabolic syndrome in younger populations has not reached consensus and different definitions exist. With central adiposity playing a central role in the metabolic syndrome, the syndrome has a strong genetic link, influenced by key environmental factors that promote excess nutrition and physical inactivity. Two components of the metabolic syndrome, type 2 diabetes and obesity, are increasingly observed in children and adolescents [36, 65] and these are believed to drive the onset of MetS [21, 32]. Indeed, prospective data has shown that excess adiposity and metabolic abnormalities in pediatric populations can result in adverse cardiometabolic profiles in adulthood [49, 81]. The Bogalusa Heart Study showed that childhood obesity tracks into adulthood [29]. Furthermore, longitudinal evidence has shown that the presence of overweight/obesity and/or metabolic abnormality at age 9-24 years predicts an increased risk of metabolic syndrome, type 2 diabetes mellitus and adverse cardiovascular outcomes 21-25 years later [47]. The problem of excess adiposity with attendant insulin resistance in adolescents is now resulting in highly invasive bariatric surgery procedures [24]. Despite these surgeries demonstrating a significant reduction in MetS prevalence from 27% to 2% [50], this treatment strategy remains controversial. Alternative treatments include targeting lifestyle behavior modification. However, success of these types of interventions can only occur once a better understanding of all contributory factors, and the extent to which they are involved, has been determined. The focus of this review is to highlight and discuss the most recent evidence surrounding factors that contribute to the onset and progression of two closely related, and increasingly prevalent, diseases in childhood (obesity and insulin resistance), which are major drivers of the global epidemic of pediatric MetS.

2. Literature Search

We searched PubMed database using the following search terms: 'metabolic syndrome' AND 'children' 'adolescent' 'pediatric'. Filters for age (0-18 years), human research and English language were applied and we restricted the search to highlight articles published in the last five years (2011-2016). Our search revealed a total of 420 articles, which were subsequently examined based on relevance to the current review. Further, we also reviewed and included relevant articles from reference sections of identified manuscripts as well as other known literature deemed pertinent to the review.

3. The Contribution of Genetics and Epigenetics upon the Risk of Obesity

It was recently purported that 10% of obesity cases can be explained by genetics and that 90% are attributable to environmental factors (discussed in later sections) [78]. Whilst the embryo develops in the intrauterine environment, multiple maternal genetic and lifestyle factors can predispose the fetus to later obesity [74]. Furthermore, interactions between the environment and genes following birth, has been linked to Deoxyribonucleic Acid (DNA) methylation alterations [74]. For example, monozygotic twins are identical, epigenetically, in the early stages of life. Progressively, however, alterations to the genetic distribution of 5-metylcytosine DNA have been noted as well as changes in histone acetylation [74]. This suggests that exposure to differing environmental stimuli may result in distinguishable genetic features. MicroRNAs are involved in the regulation of epigenetics. The influence of nutrition upon epigenetics has been previously highlighted involving methyl-group metabolism. During important developmental periods, ingestion of foods containing choline, methionine and folate, can alter DNA and histone methylation [80]. This results in chronic alterations to gene expression and the epigenetics that may predispose children to obesity later in life [80].

Oxidative stress is common in the pathogenesis of metabolic disorders and may contribute to the development of cardiovascular disease and type 2 diabetes. However, the precise role of antioxidant enzymes in the prevention of metabolic diseases is not completely understood. A recent study examined the role of Paraoxonase 1 (PON1) polymorphism (Q192R) in relation to insulin resistance in 117 children (6-12 years old) [2]. Q192R genotypes were characterized and the genotype of each sample was determined, generating three allelic clusters: QQ, QR and RR. Insulin resistance was derived using the homeostasis model assessment (HOMA-IR). An association between the polymorphism in those with the RR genotype and insulin resistance ($\geq 95^{th}$ percentile) (odds ratio [OR] = 4.55; 95% confidence intervals [CI]: 1.21-18.53) was observed. An increased risk was shown for RR carriers compared to other genotypes (OR = 6.38, p

< 0.01) [2]. Other recent genetic studies have highlighted the potential influence of polymorphisms upon metabolic health in pediatric populations [53, 77]. Despite growing evidence in the field of genetics and its link to hormone regulation, the importance of maternal health as a contributor to MetS in children has received much attention.

4. The Importance of Maternal Health in Relation to the Growth, Development and Metabolic Profile of the Offspring

Maternal health has been highlighted as a key factor for the health and development of offspring in the intrauterine environment [26]. A recent study, which examined data from 937 women and their offspring, examined the prospective relationships between fasting glucose levels during pregnancy upon multiple outcomes of the offspring's development from birth to 3 years [4]. A positive relationship was observed between gestational fasting glucose level and birth weight ($\beta = 0.17$, $p < 0.001$). Obesity in mothers before pregnancy, although self-reported, was positively associated with conditional growth in standardized BMI of the infant between birth and 1-year ($\beta = 0.10$, $p = 0.018$), birth to 18 months ($\beta = 0.11$, $p = 0.024$), birth to 2 years ($\beta = 0.14$, $p = 0.002$) as well as at 3 years ($\beta = 0.19$, $p < 0.001$), suggesting a dose-response association [4]. This study highlights the importance of maternal health in relation to subsequent growth and development of the offspring. Gestational diabetes, even when less severe, has been linked to larger birth weights and large-for-gestational age (LGA) when compared to mothers with normal glucose tolerance [43].

Further support for the importance of maternal health, even prior to conception, relating to subsequent cardiometabolic risk in the offspring has been shown. Project Viva, which recruited 1,090 mother-child pairs, demonstrated that each 5-unit increase in maternal BMI pre-pregnancy was associated with a 0.92 kg increase in total fat and 0.39 kg trunk fat in the offspring at birth. Each 5 kg of weight gained during pregnancy was positively and significantly associated with greater total and trunk adiposity (determined using dual x-ray absorptiometry) in the offspring, after adjustment [64]. Whilst mothers with gestational diabetes and pre-pregnancy obesity are show to be more likely to deliver offspring that are LGA, the negative consequences associated with LGA have been shown to persist well into childhood [30]. The long-term consequences of children born LGA include imbalances in glucose homeostasis with higher insulin resistance pre-pubertally compared to normal for gestational age counterparts [30].

Clearly, maternal health, both before and during pregnancy, has important implications for the future metabolic profile of the offspring. The mother's role in the health and development of their offspring is undisputable, including decisions about feeding methods from birth. Recent evidence has supported a link between breastfeeding and the future cardiometabolic health of the offspring. The large prospective study of 727 children, followed from birth until four years of age examined the impact of three different methods of feeding at three months as well as breastfeeding duration. Compared to children exclusively or predominantly breastfed at three months, those who were not breastfed had significantly higher mean BMI, and higher total cholesterol levels. Furthermore, children breastfed for less than three months compared to those breastfed for more than 12 months had a 0.44 increase in mean BMI at age four years [66]. This study highlights the long-term benefits of breastfeeding upon the future metabolic health of children, although there are several considerations. Breastfeeding is usually obtained from maternal reports and could be subject to social desirability bias. The use of objective measures for determining excess adiposity and adipose distribution in relation to feeding methods during infancy in relation to childhood obesity is preferable. Future studies in this area now require longer follow up given that the mean increase of 0.44 BMI over a four-year period is unlikely to be clinically relevant.

Although these studies demonstrate the importance of maternal health and early decisions about feeding during infancy that may predispose children to insulin resistance and obesity, exposure to the external environment and negative health behaviours during childhood and adolescence provide additional clues about factors that support the progression of chronic conditions associated with MetS.

5. The Contribution of Negative Health Behaviours in Relation to Obesity and Insulin Resistance in Children and Adolescents

Repeated exposure to negative health behaviours observed in childhood has been consistently linked to the subsequent practice of unhealthy lifestyle behaviours. A clear example of this is the contribution of parental obesity when investigating childhood obesity, given that this is one of the strongest predictors [57]. At a translational level, negative health habits of parents are commonly mirrored in their offspring. We will now review and discuss the contribution of a series of behaviours that are key for optimal metabolic health and body weight homeostasis in children and adolescents.

5.1. Sleep

The importance of achieving a balance between sleep and wakefulness was noted at least four decades ago in the Alameda County Study [11]. The study emphasized seven social and psychological aspects in relation to health and longevity, one of which was sleep duration [11]. This advice is not restricted to adults but also applicable to children and adolescents, with different age groups requiring different sleep quantities. More recently, sleep and has been recognized as a supplementary lifestyle factor, important for health and longevity [8, 9]. Sleep is crucial in childhood and contributes to healthy physical and neural development, yet sleep problems are common in pediatrics. The impact of insufficient sleep or poor quality sleep in pediatric populations has been extensively examined with findings consistently reporting associations between sub-optimal sleep features and increased BMI as well as insulin resistance and type 2 diabetes mellitus [40] [3, 42, 55, 73] [6]. A recent study showed that sleeping 7-9 hours had a protective effect on MetS in adolescent (OR = 0.38, 95% CI: 0.15-0.94) [25]. Mechanistic explanations for the association between sleep and metabolic abnormalities have been linked to alterations in metabolic hormones related to hunger and appetite. Not meeting individual sleep requirements can influence energy balance and may result in behaviours that promote obesity such as physical inactivity and unhealthy food intake (discussed in later sections).

The focus of attention between sleep and metabolic dysfunction has shifted with more attention now concentrating on sleep architecture. Sleep architecture (sleep staging) in relation to glucose metabolism has been explored in children and adolescents, with an initial focus on those with obesity [28, 46]. A recent study investigated the effect of sleep staging upon glucose tolerance, insulin sensitivity and pancreatic β-cell function in children and adolescents (n = 118; mean age 13.1 years; 45% boys) [82]. Sleep outcomes were assessed using the gold standard measure (polysomnography) for one-night and a 2-hour oral glucose tolerance test was administered on the subsequent morning. The amount of time spent in slow wave sleep (SWS) was significantly and positively associated with insulin sensitivity. Conversely, the amount of time spent in light sleep (stage 1) was negatively associated with insulin sensitivity. The study findings found further support for a positive linear association between sleep duration and glucose tolerance [82].

The first study to examine the effect of experimental sleep manipulation upon insulin resistance in lean adolescents was conducted by Klingenberg and colleagues [45]. This randomized crossover study assessed 21 healthy males (mean age 16.8 years), subjecting them to three nights of either short (four hours time in bed) or long (nine hours time in bed) sleep opportunity. Insulin resistance was determined from pre and post-prandial levels of glucose and insulin at the end of each sleep condition. Whilst they observed no change in glucose level between the two sleep conditions, insulin resistance significantly increased by 65% following sleep restriction compared to the nine-hour sleep opportunity [45]. Interestingly, adolescents with insulin resistance compared to those without, have been shown to have a reduced amount of stage 2 and 3 sleep (light and deep sleep, respectively). Deep sleep, also known as slow wave sleep, is known for its restorative properties including cell repair. Thus, a reduced amount of slow wave sleep activity is likely to produce downstream effects on hormone secretion and metabolic function. Notably, sleep-disordered breathing (SDB) is associated with disruptions to sleep architecture and has become increasingly recognized in pediatric populations to OSA diagnosis in children). Interestingly, more severe obstructive sleep apena (OSA), a SDB condition, has also been linked to greater insulin resistance and elevated glucose levels in children [70]. Given previous reports of a close relationship between OSA and MetS in adolescents [68] and the increasing prevalence of these conditions in pediatric populations, SDB is an important consideration for future research studies in this area.

There are many features of sleep to be considered. For example, sleep timing and circadian rhythmicity are essential sleep parameters to scrutinize. Delays in circadian sleep-wake patterns are common during adolescence due to a combination of pubertal transition and psychosocial factors. A recent study examined the effect of circadian preference upon BMI in a large sample (n = 511) of young adolescents (aged 11-13 years) and found that those with a later preference had significantly greater BMI z-scores ($\beta = 0.51$, $p < 0.01$) [8]. Furthermore, the study also revealed those with later preferences had poorer dietary habits [8]; thus alterations to sleep and circadian imbalance have the potential to disrupt energy homeostasis and well as appetite regulating hormones [38], which in turn, may result in weight gain and insulin resistance.

5.2. Diet

The importance of a healthy diet and optimum nutrition has been consistently emphasized in recent decades through national campaigns following recognition of poor dietary habits. This has been highlighted as a result of exposure to an 'obesogenic' environment. Rapid changes and increased exposure to food availability, including processed, ready-made and fast foods, has been purported to influence dietary intake. These modified foods tend to have higher sugar, salt and calorie contents. Over-consumption of these food items is likely to result in positive energy, which in turn, promotes obesity and/or insulin resistance if levels of energy expenditure are insufficient to counteract energy imbalance. Campaigns have aimed at educating individuals to improve dietary behaviours have included information about healthy portion sizes, reducing sugary food/beverage intake and increasing healthy food selection (consumption of five portions of fruit/vegetables per day). Despite raised awareness and dietary guidelines, recent prospective evidence from a birth cohort in Australia revealed that, on average, less than half of the total sample met the requirements at either 14 or 17 years of age [17]. Moreover, further support for a significant negative linear association between meeting dietary guidelines and insulin resistance was reported [17]. The most recent evidence surrounding the contribution of diet in relation to MetS in children has focused on examining diet types (vegetarian and Mediterranean), specific foods (white rice) and macronutrients (saturated fat), each discussed in turn.

The beneficial effects of a Mediterranean diet upon cardiovascular health have been extensively reported in adults [14, 34, 35, 48, 67, 79] although less evidence is available in pediatric populations. In particular, the effect of a Mediterranean-style diet in children at high risk of MetS, has been recently explored, revealing positive results [76]. Children and adolescents (n = 49; mean age 11 years) attending a family medical center were included if they had BMI $\geq 95^{th}$ percentile as well as any other feature of MetS, according to the International Diabetes Federation (IDF) criteria [1]. Of the total sample, 24 were randomized to receive education and instructions to follow a Mediterranean-style diet and the remaining 25 followed a standard diet for 16 weeks, supported by parents [76]. Anthropometric measures (height, weight, waist and circumference, and bioelectrical impedance), blood pressure and fasting blood samples were recorded/obtained at baseline and at the end of the 16-week dietary intervention. Food recall (24-hour) was used to quantify calorie, macro and micronutrient content every three weeks throughout the intervention period. Those in the Mediterranean diet group had a significant mean reduction in BMI, fat mass, lean mass, as well as glucose, total cholesterol, low-density lipoprotein (LDL) and triglyceride levels at the end of the intervention compared to baseline. An increase in levels of high-density lipoprotein (HDL) was also observed in the same group. Furthermore, the number of MetS components significantly decreased from baseline to the end of the 16-week intervention in those following the Mediterranean diet and meeting the criteria for MetS decreased by 45% [76]. Whilst these study results provide powerful support for promoting a Mediterranean diet, caution with interpretation of the findings is necessary. Limitations of the study include 1) small sample size; 2) individualized recommended daily calorie intake based on age and sex-specific cut points rather than basal metabolic rate; 3) relatively short intervention period with no report on compliance to the diet condition at each of the three weekly assessments; 4) between group differences were not reported, which is important given that the standard diet group also received lifestyle and dietary advice with suggested modification; 5) the differences between the two diet interventions were minimal; 6) no assessment of continued compliance to the diet or MetS monitoring beyond the study period; 7) no adjustment was performed for any potential confounders; and 8) subjective dietary measures, possibly resulting in social desirability and recall bias.

The Mediterranean diet is largely plant-based, with the exception of fish. A recent review of the literature suggests that a vegetarian diet can reduce all-cause and specific-cause mortality (cancer, cardiovascular, type 2 diabetes mellitus) [69]. The beneficial effect of fruit and vegetable consumption in childhood has been prospectively assessed in relation to components of MetS by at least two groups. A large cohort (n = 2,218) of children and adolescents (aged 3-18 years at baseline), followed for ~27 years found a 14% decreased risk of developing MetS in those with a higher intake of vegetables during childhood. Furthermore, the study also revealed that higher vegetable consumption in childhood decreased the risk of high blood pressure (OR = 0.88, 95% CI: 0.80-0.98) and elevated triglycerides (OR = 0.88, 95% CI: 0.79-0.99) at the time measured during adulthood [41]. The Child-Adolescent Blood Pressure Study reported similar findings following assessment of food intake derived from a 106-item food frequency questionnaire administered to 1,764 children and adolescents (aged 6-19 years) [56]. A Registered Dietitian condensed food items into seven categories: grains, nuts, fruits, vegetables, dairy, meats and low-nutrient-dense foods. Those in the highest quartile of grains, vegetables, nuts and low-nutrient-dense foods consumption had a reduced risk of being overweight (BMI > 85th percentile), where corresponding ORs (95% CIs) were 0.59 (0.41-0.83), 0.67 (0.48-0.94), 0.60 (0.43-0.85) and 0.43 (0.29-0.63), respectively. Whilst the categories of nuts and vegetable consumption are consistent with other study findings [41, 62], the most surprising finding was that of low-nutrient-dense foods which was shown as a protective factor for overweight. The authors explained this by suggesting that consumption of foods in this category may have been under-reported, possibly due to social acceptance [56], which may be a common issue when assessing dietary habits.

A balanced diet involves the incorporation of multiple macronutrients. Carbohydrate content and glycemic load have been recent focuses in nutritional research. Efforts have been made to examine the effect of white rice intake in adolescents upon MetS and its components, in populations where rice is a staple food. Data obtained from the Fourth Korea National Health and Nutrition Examination Survey, during 2007-2009, was used [72]. Information was available from 2,209 adolescents (aged 10-18 years) and features of MetS were objectively acquired. Diet was assessed using 24-hour food recall and white rice consumption was divided into quartiles. Analysis was performed according to gender. Girls in the highest quartile of white rice consumption had greater insulin resistance ($p = 0.005$) and lower HDL-cholesterol ($p < 0.001$), compared to the other three quartiles. Girls in the two upper quartiles of white rice intake were more likely to meet the criteria for MetS ($p = 0.003$) [72]. These findings were not found in boys and explanation for this is possibly related to differences in insulin-like growth factors and/or sex hormones during pubertal transition. However, gender differences have been observed in multiple adult studies [23, 59, 60] suggesting that women with high white rice/carbohydrate/glycemic load have more adverse metabolic profiles, compared to men. The authors purported that high consumption of white rice may result in altered glucose metabolism and dyslipidemia [72]. The macronutrient breakdown and proportion of each category (fats, carbohydrates, protein) is clearly important and has been the recent focus of a randomized controlled trial.

Nupponen and colleagues report on findings from the Special Turku Coronary Risk Factor Intervention Project (STRIP) [61]. The trial aimed to reduce children's intake of saturated fat through dietary counseling and to examine the effectiveness of the program upon preventing later atherosclerosis. The study recruited five-month old infants and parents (1990-1992). At six months of age, 1,062 infants and their parents were randomly assigned to either the intervention ($n = 540$) or control condition ($n = 522$). The intervention group received individualized dietary counseling every two years until the infant reached 20 years of age. The primary aim of the intervention was to replaced saturated fat with unsaturated fat in the diet of the child, which was supported by counseling and nutritional advice. Counseling was parent-focused until the child was 7 years old. Beyond this age, the advice gradually increased to be more child-focused. Food records were used to make suggestions about methods for improving diet. The control group was also seen every two years and received basic health education as part of standard Finnish care. Individual components of MetS were measured at study visits when the child was 15-20 years old. As previously described, there is no consensus on universal criteria for MetS in pediatric populations therefore the study applied five separate definitions. This resulted in a range (6.0-7.5%) for meeting a diagnosis of MetS in the intervention group and 10-14% in the control group between age 15-20 years. The long-term risk of developing MetS in the intervention group was significantly lower (relative risk [RR] = 0.59, 95% CI: 0.40-0.88) compared to the control group. There was further evidence to support the efficacy of the intervention for individual components of MetS including a decreased risk of hypertension where RR = 0.83 95% CI: 0.70-0.99 and high triglycerides in males (RR = 0.71, 95% CI: 0.52-0.98). The authors concluded that repeated dietary advice, targeted at reducing saturated fat intake during childhood, reduces the risk of MetS and its associated features [61].

Undoubtedly, diet is a crucial lifestyle component for ensuring a healthy metabolic profile later on in life. Many studies that examine the relationships between lifestyle factors believed to predict MetS and its features, do not adjust for the effect of diet, which is a major concern and should be addressed in future studies. Parental involvement and education concerning diet, and other contributory yet modifiable behaviours, during early parenthood and beyond may be necessary for optimizing the future health and longevity of the offspring.

5.3. Screen Time

Over the last decade, there has been a surge in the availability and accessibility of electronic devices. Portable equivalents of what used to be static media (television, telephones, computers and gaming consoles) are now increasingly available and ownership has increased amongst children and adolescents. Engaging in the use of these devices has been purported to promote unhealthy lifestyles by increasing levels of sedentariness (see next section). Other consequences include limitation of face-to-face interactions, resulting in social isolation/loneliness, lowered self-confidence and addiction [12], which has been prospectively linked to circadian disruption in pediatrics [18]. Children, from a young age, may be permitted and encouraged to use electronic media communication devices with tablet holders now available to secure onto pushchairs. Whilst there are many benefits of these devices, concerns about the impact upon health have been raised. Early data from the National Health And Nutrition Examination Survey (NHANES) revealed a dose-dependent association between the amount of daily screen time (television and computer use) and MetS in 12-19 year olds [54]. After adjustment for physical activity level, the risk of MetS was more than three-fold for adolescents spending five hours per day on screens compared to those using screens for one-hour or less [54]. These findings are consistent with more recent evidence from the same survey, conducted in Korean children and adolescents. Compared to the lowest quartile of screen time use (≤16 hours per week), those in the highest quartile (≥35 hours per week) were more than twice as likely to meet the criteria for MetS after adjustment (OR = 2.23 95% CI: 1.02-4.86) [44].

Progressive technology use with increasing age in adolescents has been associated with increased levels of sedentariness/physical inactivity [20, 37], possibly displacing activities involving greater energy expenditure. Persistent use can therefore result in obesity development. In combination, obesity onset may be exacerbated through over-consumption of foods that are high in calories, fat and sugar. Some have shown that exposure to advertisements marketing unhealthy foods trigger intake of these food items [27, 31], which in turn, can promote weight gain and subsequent obesity. Paradoxically, preliminary evidence has shown that video games involving physical activity can enhance weight loss in overweight/obese children [19, 52, 75]. The relationship between technology use and obesity and/or insulin resistance is, however, convoluted.

The complex interactions between technology use and childhood obesity/metabolic dysfunction may be mediated by sleep [7], food/beverage intake [20] and physical inactivity [20]. In a study of 738 young adolescent (11-13 years old), the use of six different types of technology at bedtime was examined in relation to eight sleep features [5]. More frequent use of all technology before bedtime was associated with multiple adverse effects on sleep [5]. Explanations for technology use resulting in adverse sleep outcomes are mental excitation/stimulation and exposure to blue light, emitted from electronic devices, which can suppress melatonin release and delay sleep onset. The same group examined the mediating effect of sleep duration upon the established relationship between technology use and adolescent BMI [7]. Bedtime use of all four technologies assessed was related to shorter sleep duration [7]. A negative association was also observed between sleep duration and BMI (β = -0.40, $p < 0.01$), consistent with other studies. Sleep duration was recognized as a mediator of the relationship between portable types of technology (mobile telephones and computers) and BMI [7]. This suggests the direct association between screen-time and obesity in children/adolescents is complex, requiring consideration of multiple factors and lifestyle behaviours.

The use of technology in teenagers is particularly problematic given that this group commonly experience circadian phase delay during pubertal transition. This results in later bed times with more free time in the evening, which may be consumed by engaging with devices. Recent evidence has shown that 94% of adolescent boys and 87% of girls spent more than 2 hours, daily, engaging in screen-based activities [20]. A concomitant behavior is the consumption of caffeinated beverages and/or sugar-sweetened beverages in adolescents [15, 20, 23]. Both of these behaviors, whether examined singularly or in combination, have been linked to poorer sleep outcomes and/or obesity [5-7, 16, 51], and are also likely to influence metabolic regulation. Consideration should be given to this emerging area of study, particularly as both technology use and consumption of sugar-dense beverages with low nutritional content, have been shown to increase with age in pediatric populations [37, 51].

Most recent evidence from a large prospective cohort of children, suggests that interventions aimed at reducing screen time and sedentariness in children at risk of obesity, may help to alleviate the risk of MetS development [39]. This recommendation reinforces the notion that modification to multiple lifestyle factors, which are known drivers of MetS and its individual components, need to be tackled in a timely manner, one of which is sedentariness.

5.4. Sedentariness

Low levels of physical activity reflect sedentariness and long, persistent episodes can result in positive energy and subsequent obesity and/or insulin resistance, particularly when combined with other negative related health behaviours. The contribution of energy expenditure upon metabolic health is well recognized. One of the largest studies to date to examine the association between levels of sedentariness and central obesity was conducted in 124,113 Greek school-aged children (9.9 ± 1.1 years old, 51% male). A seven-day recall questionnaire was administered which asked about diet and physical activity habits and anthropometric measures were obtained [33]. Central obesity was prevalent in 33.4% of the sample and revealed significant associations between the condition and frequent (at least four times per week) breakfast consumption (OR = 0.72 95% CI: 0.69-0.75), habitual snack consumption both at midday and the afternoon (OR = 0.70 95% CI: 0.67-0.74) and high levels of sedentariness, defined as participation in sedentary activities ≥4 times per week, OR = 1.10 (95% CI: 1.07-1.14). The authors concluded that emphasis should be placed on regular meal consumption and reducing levels of sedentariness [33].

A recent cross-sectional study examined the contribution of diet and physical activity levels upon the metabolic profiles of 667 Chilean adolescents (16-17 years old; 52.2% male) [13]. Of the total sample 9.5% met the criteria for MetS. Physical activity was measured using a validated, standardized questionnaire with scores ranging 0-10. Physical inactivity was determined using a cut point of ≤3 and was recognized as a major contributor to MetS, where OR = 2.9 (95% CI: 1.1-7.7) [13]. Whilst the importance of consistent physical activity in childhood can be emphasized for later metabolic and cardiovascular health, the school environment may inadvertently impede adequate levels of activity.

Sedentariness is a particular problem in the academic environment [22] where children are required to remain seated throughout the majority of lessons. Findings from a recently published randomized controlled trial (RCT) aiming to address this concern reported positive, albeit minimal, improvements to obesity in children [58]. The study compared findings of the intervention group, where children performed one daily physical activity session of one-hour during school time, to the control group, which undertook two physical activity sessions per week over a four-year timeframe [58]. Mean BMI and proportion of childhood overweight were similar across the two groups at baseline. At the end of the four-year intervention period, a larger proportion of those in the intervention group were between the 10-90th percentile for BMI compared to the control group, 87% versus 78%, respectively. However, this difference was not statistically significant ($p = 0.13$). Childhood overweight (BMI >90th percentile) was consistently lower in the intervention group compared to the control group across all annual assessments. However, the authors present no formal statistical analysis for these relationships and it therefore remains unclear if these findings were statistically significant or not. The high withdrawal rate of overweight/obese children (44%) across the total sample is also likely to have influenced the findings [58]. Whilst this is the most recent RCT to report on the effectiveness of overcoming sedentariness in an academic setting, additional studies need to be performed in this area. The importance of an active lifestyle requires educating both children and parents to ensure that the appropriate level of support, attention, application and reinforcement is provided, outside of the academic environment.

6. Recommendations for Tackling MetS in Pediatrics

Educational interventions in mothers, before, during, and beyond pregnancy appear to be paramount for reducing the risk of later obesity in the offspring. Parents are major role models to their children and early, persistent exposure to healthy lifestyle practices ensure that these are more likely to be adopted by the offspring. Moreover, modification of parental behaviors influence the child's and has been shown to reflect similar behavioral change [71]. Addressing, and attempting to reverse, negative health-related behaviors at an early age are necessary to encourage healthy lifestyles and minimize the onset of metabolic disorders. Modification of unhealthy lifestyle habits, that are becoming more prevalent in contemporary society (later bedtimes, exposure to electronic media at night-time, consumption of energy/caffeinated drinks, sedentariness and poor diet), should be specifically targeted and minimized wherever possible. Successful interventions are likely to require parental involvement, which could help to curb the rising prevalence of childhood obesity, insulin resistance and MetS. Methods to reduce increasing levels of sedentariness in children and adolescents, both in the home and academic environment, are urgently required.

7. Conclusions

Maternal health, even prior to conception, plays a crucial role in the growth, development and future metabolic profile of the offspring. The metabolic health of women should be investigated and advice provided to those in the planning stages of pregnancy. Weight loss in those with excess adiposity before conceiving should be targeted. Excessive weight gain during pregnancy should be managed in an attempt to improve the future cardiometabolic outcomes of the offspring. Parental involvement, (particularly the mother) at all stages of an intervention aimed at children, is likely to be fundamental to the success of future trials. Further study of epigenetics and the relevance of specific polymorphisms is also required to better understand the influence the metabolic profile of children and adolescents. Sleep optimization and education about the importance of this behavior, which is currently overlooked, may be a promising tool and contribute to healthy metabolic regulation in pediatric populations. Clearly, a holistic, multi-disciplinary approach targeting multiple health-related behaviors is now required.

References

[1] Alberti G, Zimmet P, Shaw J, Bloomgarden Z, Kaufman F, Silink M, et al. Type 2 diabetes in the young: the evolving epidemic: the international diabetes federation consensus workshop. Diabetes Care. 2004;27 (7):1798-811.

[2] Alegria-Torres JA, Garcia-Dominguez ML, Cruz M, Aradillas-Garcia C. Q192R polymorphism of paraoxonase 1 gene associated with insulin resistance in Mexican children. Arch Med Res. 2015;46 (1):78-83.

[3] Androutsos O, Moschonis G, Mavrogianni C, Roma-Giannikou E, Chrousos GP, Kanaka-Gantenbein C, et al. Identification of lifestyle patterns, including sleep deprivation, associated with insulin resistance in children: the Healthy Growth Study. Eur J Clin Nutr. 2014;68 (3):344-9.

[4] Aris IM, Soh SE, Tint MT, Saw SM, Rajadurai VS, Godfrey KM, et al. Associations of gestational glycemia and prepregnancy adiposity with offspring growth and adiposity in an Asian population. Am J Clin Nutr. 2015;102 (5):1104-12.

[5] Arora T, Broglia E, Thomas GN, Taheri S. Associations between specific technologies and adolescent sleep quantity, sleep quality, and parasomnias. Sleep Med. 2014;15 (2):240-7.

[6] Arora T, Hosseini-Araghi M, Bishop J, Yao GL, Thomas GN, Taheri S. The complexity of obesity in U.K. adolescents: relationships with quantity and type of technology, sleep duration and quality, academic performance and aspiration. Pediatr Obes. 2013;8 (5):358-66.

[7] Arora T, Hussain S, Hubert Lam KB, Lily Yao G, Neil Thomas G, Taheri S. Exploring the complex pathways among specific types of technology, self-reported sleep duration and body mass index in UK adolescents. Int J Obes (Lond). 2013;37 (9):1254-60.

[8] Arora T, Taheri S. Associations among late chronotype, body mass index and dietary behaviors in young adolescents. Int J Obes (Lond). 2015;39 (1):39-44.

[9] Arora T, Taheri S. Sleep Optimization and Diabetes Control: A Review of the Literature. Diabetes Ther. 2015;6 (4):425-68.

[10] Arora T. Sleep Doesn't Waste Time, It's Good for the Waist Line. Sleep. 2015;38 (8):1159-60.

[11] Belloc NB, Breslow L. Relationship of physical health status and health practices. Prev Med. 1972;1 (3):409-21.

[12] Boniel-Nissim M, Lenzi M, Zsiros E, de Matos MG, Gommans R, Harel-Fisch Y, et al. International trends in electronic media communication among 11- to 15-year-olds in 30 countries from 2002 to 2010: association with ease of communication with friends of the opposite sex. Eur J Public Health. 2015;25 Suppl 2:41-5.

[13] Burrows R, Correa-Burrows P, Reyes M, Blanco E, Albala C, Gahagan S. High cardiometabolic risk in healthy Chilean adolescents: associations with anthropometric, biological and lifestyle factors. Public Health Nutr. 2016;19 (3):486-93.

[14] Buscemi S, Nicolucci A, Mattina A, Rosafio G, Massenti FM, Lucisano G, et al. Association of dietary patterns with insulin resistance and clinically silent carotid atherosclerosis in apparently healthy people. Eur J Clin Nutr. 2013;67 (12):1284-90.

[15] Calamaro CJ, Yang K, Ratcliffe S, Chasens ER. Wired at a young age: the effect of caffeine and technology on sleep duration and body mass index in school-aged children. J Pediatr Health Care. 2012;26 (4):276-82.

[16] Centers for Disease C, Prevention. Beverage consumption among high school students — United States, 2010. MMWR Morb Mortal Wkly Rep. 2011;60 (23):778-80.

[17] Chan She Ping-Delfos WL, Beilin LJ, Oddy WH, Burrows S, Mori TA. Use of the Dietary Guideline Index to assess cardiometabolic risk in adolescents. Br J Nutr. 2015;113 (11):1741-52.

[18] Chen YL, Gau SS. Sleep problems and internet addiction among children and adolescents: a longitudinal study. J Sleep Res. 2016;25 (4):458-65.

[19] Christison A, Khan HA. Exergaming for health: a community-based pediatric weight management program using active video gaming. Clin Pediatr (Phila). 2012;51 (4):382-8.

[20] Christofaro DG, De Andrade SM, Mesas AE, Fernandes RA, Farias Junior JC. Higher screen time is associated with overweight, poor dietary habits and physical inactivity in Brazilian adolescents, mainly among girls. Eur J Sport Sci. 2016;16 (4):498-506.

[21] Cornier MA, Dabelea D, Hernandez TL, Lindstrom RC, Steig AJ, Stob NR, et al. The metabolic syndrome. Endocr Rev. 2008;29 (7):777-822.

[22] De Decker E, De Craemer M, De Bourdeaudhuij I, Wijndaele K, Duvinage K, Androutsos O, et al. Influencing factors of sedentary behavior in European preschool settings: an exploration through focus groups with teachers. J Sch Health. 2013;83 (9):654-61.

[23] Demissie Z, Lowry R, Eaton DK, Park S, Kann L. Electronic media and beverage intake among United States high school students–2010. J Nutr Educ Behav. 2013;45 (6):756-60.

[24] Dillard BE, 3rd, Gorodner V, Galvani C, Holterman M, Browne A, Gallo A, et al. Initial experience with the adjustable gastric band in morbidly obese US adolescents and recommendations for further investigation. J Pediatr Gastroenterol Nutr. 2007;45 (2):240-6.

[25] Fadzlina AA, Harun F, Nurul Haniza MY, Al Sadat N, Murray L, Cantwell MM, et al. Metabolic syndrome among 13 year old adolescents: prevalence and risk factors. BMC Public Health. 2014;14 Suppl 3:S7.

[26] Faienza MF, Wang DQ, Fruhbeck G, Garruti G, Portincasa P. The dangerous link between childhood and adulthood predictors of obesity and metabolic syndrome. Intern Emerg Med. 2016;11 (2):175-82.

[27] Falbe J, Willett WC, Rosner B, Gortmaker SL, Sonneville KR, Field AE. Longitudinal relations of television, electronic games, and digital versatile discs with changes in diet in adolescents. Am J Clin Nutr. 2014;100 (4):1173-81.

[28] Flint J, Kothare SV, Zihlif M, Suarez E, Adams R, Legido A, et al. Association between inadequate sleep and insulin resistance in obese children. J Pediatr. 2007;150 (4):364-9.

[29] Freedman DS, Mei Z, Srinivasan SR, Berenson GS, Dietz WH. Cardiovascular risk factors and excess adiposity among overweight children and adolescents: the Bogalusa Heart Study. J Pediatr. 2007;150 (1):12-7 e2.

[30] Giapros VI, Challa AS, Cholevas VI, Evagelidou EN, Bairaktari ET, Andronikou SK. Vitamin D, parathormone, and insulin resistance in children born large for gestational age. J Pediatr Endocrinol Metab. 2014;27 (11-12):1145-50.

[31] Giese H, Konig LM, Taut D, Ollila H, Baban A, Absetz P, et al. Exploring the association between television advertising of healthy and unhealthy foods, self-control, and food intake in three European countries. Appl Psychol Health Well Being. 2015;7 (1):41-62.

[32] Goff DC, Jr., Lloyd-Jones DM, Bennett G, Coady S, D'Agostino RB, Sr., Gibbons R, et al. 2013 ACC/AHA guideline on the assessment of cardiovascular risk: a report of the American College of Cardiology/American Heart Association Task Force on Practice Guidelines. J Am Coll Cardiol. 2014;63 (25 Pt B):2935-59.

[33] Grigorakis DA, Georgoulis M, Psarra G, Tambalis KD, Panagiotakos DB, Sidossis LS. Prevalence and lifestyle determinants of central obesity in children. Eur J Nutr. 2016;55 (5):1923-31.

[34] Grosso G, Marventano S, Galvano F, Pajak A, Mistretta A. Factors associated with metabolic syndrome in a mediterranean population: role of caffeinated beverages. J Epidemiol. 2014;24 (4):327-33.

[35] Grosso G, Pajak A, Mistretta A, Marventano S, Raciti T, Buscemi S, et al. Protective role of the Mediterranean diet on several cardiovascular risk factors: evidence from Sicily, southern Italy. Nutr Metab Cardiovasc Dis. 2014;24 (4):370-7.

[36] Han JC, Lawlor DA, Kimm SY. Childhood obesity. Lancet. 2010;375 (9727):1737-48.

[37] Hardy LL, Bass SL, Booth ML. Changes in sedentary behavior among adolescent girls: a 2.5-year prospective cohort study. J Adolesc Health. 2007;40 (2):158-65.

[38] Hart CN, Carskadon MA, Considine RV, Fava JL, Lawton J, Raynor HA, et al. Changes in children's sleep duration on food intake, weight, and leptin. Pediatrics. 2013;132 (6):e1473-80.

[39] Henderson M, Benedetti A, Barnett TA, Mathieu ME, Deladoey J, Gray-Donald K. Influence of Adiposity, Physical Activity, Fitness, and Screen Time on Insulin Dynamics Over 2 Years in Children. JAMA Pediatr. 2016;170 (3):227-35.

[40] Hitze B, Bosy-Westphal A, Bielfeldt F, Settler U, Plachta-Danielzik S, Pfeuffer M, et al. Determinants and impact of sleep duration in children and adolescents: data of the Kiel Obesity Prevention Study. Eur J Clin Nutr. 2009;63 (6):739-46.

[41] Jaaskelainen P, Magnussen CG, Pahkala K, Mikkila V, Kahonen M, Sabin MA, et al. Childhood nutrition in predicting metabolic syndrome in adults: the cardiovascular risk in Young Finns Study. Diabetes Care. 2012;35 (9):1937-43.

[42] Javaheri S, Storfer-Isser A, Rosen CL, Redline S. Association of short and long sleep durations with insulin sensitivity in adolescents. J Pediatr. 2011;158 (4):617-23.

[43] Kanai Y, Kamoda T, Saito M, Fujiyama S, Nishimura K, Iwabuchi A, et al. Cord blood insulin-like growth factor (IGF)-1, IGF-binding proteins and adiponectin, and birth size in offspring of women with mild gestational diabetes. Early Hum Dev. 2016;93:39-42.

[44] Kang HT, Lee HR, Shim JY, Shin YH, Park BJ, Lee YJ. Association between screen time and metabolic syndrome in children and adolescents in Korea: the 2005 Korean National Health and Nutrition Examination Survey. Diabetes Res Clin Pract. 2010;89 (1):72-8.

[45] Klingenberg L, Chaput JP, Holmback U, Visby T, Jennum P, Nikolic M, et al. Acute Sleep Restriction Reduces Insulin Sensitivity in Adolescent Boys. Sleep. 2013;36 (7):1085-90.

[46] Koren D, Levitt Katz LE, Brar PC, Gallagher PR, Berkowitz RI, Brooks LJ. Sleep architecture and glucose and insulin homeostasis in obese adolescents. Diabetes Care. 2011;34 (11):2442-7.

[47] Koskinen J, Magnussen CG, Sabin MA, Kahonen M, Hutri-Kahonen N, Laitinen T, et al. Youth overweight and metabolic disturbances in predicting carotid intima-media thickness, type 2 diabetes, and metabolic syndrome in adulthood: the Cardiovascular Risk in Young Finns study. Diabetes Care. 2014;37 (7):1870-7.

[48] Kris-Etherton P, Eckel RH, Howard BV, St Jeor S, Bazzarre TL, Nutrition Committee Population Science C, et al. AHA Science Advisory: Lyon Diet Heart Study. Benefits of a Mediterranean-style, National Cholesterol Education Program/American Heart Association Step I Dietary Pattern on Cardiovascular Disease. Circulation. 2001;103 (13):1823-5.

[49] Li S, Chen W, Srinivasan SR, Xu J, Berenson GS. Relation of childhood obesity/cardiometabolic phenotypes to adult cardiometabolic profile: the Bogalusa Heart Study. Am J Epidemiol. 2012;176 Suppl 7:S142-9.

[50] Loy JJ, Youn HA, Schwack B, Kurian M, Ren Fielding C, Fielding GA. Improvement in nonalcoholic fatty liver disease and metabolic syndrome in adolescents undergoing bariatric surgery. Surg Obes Relat Dis. 2015;11 (2):442-9.

[51] Ludwig DS, Peterson KE, Gortmaker SL. Relation between consumption of sugar-sweetened drinks and childhood obesity: a prospective, observational analysis. Lancet. 2001;357 (9255):505-8.

[52] Maddison R, Foley L, Ni Mhurchu C, Jiang Y, Jull A, Prapavessis H, et al. Effects of active video games on body composition: a randomized controlled trial. Am J Clin Nutr. 2011;94 (1):156-63.

[53] Marcil V, Amre D, Seidman EG, Boudreau F, Gendron FP, Menard D, et al. Hepatocyte nuclear factor 4 alpha polymorphisms and the metabolic syndrome in French-Canadian youth. PLoS One. 2015;10 (2):e0117238.

[54] Mark AE, Janssen I. Relationship between screen time and metabolic syndrome in adolescents. J Public Health (Oxf). 2008;30 (2):153-60.

[55] Matthews KA, Dahl RE, Owens JF, Lee L, Hall M. Sleep duration and insulin resistance in healthy black and white adolescents. Sleep. 2012;35 (10):1353-8.

[56] Matthews VL, Wien M, Sabate J. The risk of child and adolescent overweight is related to types of food consumed. Nutr J. 2011;10:71.

[57] Monzani A, Rapa A, Fuiano N, Diddi G, Prodam F, Bellone S, et al. Metabolic syndrome is strictly associated with parental obesity beginning from childhood. Clin Endocrinol (Oxf). 2014;81 (1):45-51.

[58] Muller UM, Walther C, Adams V, Mende M, Adam J, Fikenzer K, et al. Long term impact of one daily unit of physical exercise at school on cardiovascular risk factors in school children. Eur J Prev Cardiol. 2016;23 (13):1444-52.

[59] Nakashima M, Sakurai M, Nakamura K, Miura K, Yoshita K, Morikawa Y, et al. Dietary glycemic index, glycemic load and blood lipid levels in middle-aged Japanese men and women. J Atheroscler Thromb. 2010;17 (10):1082-95.

[60] Nanri A, Mizoue T, Noda M, Takahashi Y, Kato M, Inoue M, et al. Rice intake and type 2 diabetes in Japanese men and women: the Japan Public Health Center-based Prospective Study. Am J Clin Nutr. 2010;92 (6):1468-77.

[61] Nupponen M, Pahkala K, Juonala M, Magnussen CG, Niinikoski H, Ronnemaa T, et al. Metabolic syndrome from adolescence to early adulthood: effect of infancy-onset dietary counseling of low saturated fat: the Special Turku Coronary Risk Factor Intervention Project (STRIP). Circulation. 2015;131 (7):605-13.

[62] O'Neil CE, Fulgoni VL, 3rd, Nicklas TA. Tree Nut consumption is associated with better adiposity measures and cardiovascular and metabolic syndrome health risk factors in U.S. Adults: NHANES 2005-2010. Nutr J. 2015;14:64.

[63] Park SH, Lee KS, Park HY. Dietary carbohydrate intake is associated with cardiovascular disease risk in Korean: analysis of the third Korea National Health and Nutrition Examination Survey (KNHANES III). Int J Cardiol. 2010;139 (3):234-40.

[64] Perng W, Gillman MW, Mantzoros CS, Oken E. A prospective study of maternal prenatal weight and offspring cardiometabolic health in midchildhood. Ann Epidemiol. 2014;24 (11):793-800 e1.

[65] Pontiroli AE. Type 2 diabetes mellitus is becoming the most common type of diabetes in school children. Acta Diabetol. 2004;41 (3):85-90.

[66] Ramirez-Silva I, Rivera JA, Trejo-Valdivia B, Martorell R, Stein AD, Romieu I, et al. Breastfeeding status at age 3 months is associated with adiposity and cardiometabolic markers at age 4 years in Mexican children. J Nutr. 2015;145 (6):1295-302.

[67] Razquin C, Martinez JA, Martinez-Gonzalez MA, Mitjavila MT, Estruch R, Marti A. A 3 years follow-up of a Mediterranean diet rich in virgin olive oil is associated with high plasma antioxidant capacity and reduced body weight gain. Eur J Clin Nutr. 2009;63 (12):1387-93.

[68] Redline S, Storfer-Isser A, Rosen CL, Johnson NL, Kirchner HL, Emancipator J, et al. Association between metabolic syndrome and sleep-disordered breathing in adolescents. Am J Respir Crit Care Med. 2007;176 (4):401-8.

[69] Sabate J, Wien M. A perspective on vegetarian dietary patterns and risk of metabolic syndrome. Br J Nutr. 2015;113 Suppl 2:S136-43.

[70] Shamsuzzaman A, Szczesniak RD, Fenchel MC, Amin RS. Glucose, insulin, and insulin resistance in normal-weight, overweight and obese children with obstructive sleep apnea. Obes Res Clin Pract. 2014;8 (6):e584-91.

[71] Skouteris H, McCabe M, Swinburn B, Newgreen V, Sacher P, Chadwick P. Parental influence and obesity prevention in pre-schoolers: a systematic review of interventions. Obes Rev. 2011;12 (5):315-28.

[72] Song S, Young Paik H, Song WO, Song Y. Metabolic syndrome risk factors are associated with white rice intake in Korean adolescent girls and boys. Br J Nutr. 2015;113 (3):479-87.

[73] Spruyt K, Molfese DL, Gozal D. Sleep duration, sleep regularity, body weight, and metabolic homeostasis in school-aged children. Pediatrics. 2011;127 (2):e345-52.

[74] Stoger R. Epigenetics and obesity. Pharmacogenomics. 2008;9 (12):1851-60.

[75] Trost SG, Sundal D, Foster GD, Lent MR, Vojta D. Effects of a pediatric weight management program with and without active video games a randomized trial. JAMA Pediatr. 2014;168 (5):407-13.

[76] Velazquez-Lopez L, Santiago-Diaz G, Nava-Hernandez J, Munoz-Torres AV, Medina-Bravo P, Torres-Tamayo M. Mediterranean-style diet reduces metabolic syndrome components in obese children and adolescents with obesity. BMC Pediatr. 2014;14:175.

[77] White MJ, Eren F, Agirbasli D, Williams SM, Agirbasli M. SHBG gene polymorphism (rs1799941) associates with metabolic syndrome in children and adolescents. PLoS One. 2015;10 (2):e0116915.

[78] Xu S, Xue Y. Pediatric obesity: Causes, symptoms, prevention and treatment. Exp Ther Med. 2016;11 (1):15-20.

[79] Yang J, Farioli A, Korre M, Kales SN. Modified Mediterranean diet score and cardiovascular risk in a North American working population. PLoS One. 2014;9 (2):e87539.

[80] Zeisel SH. Epigenetic mechanisms for nutrition determinants of later health outcomes. Am J Clin Nutr. 2009;89 (5):1488S-93S.

[81] Zhang H, Zhang T, Li S, Li Y, Hussain A, Fernandez C, et al. Long-term Impact of Childhood Adiposity on Adult Metabolic Syndrome Is Modified by Insulin Resistance: The Bogalusa Heart Study. Sci Rep. 2015;5:17885.

[82] Zhu Y, Li AM, Au CT, Kong AP, Zhang J, Wong CK, et al. Association between sleep architecture and glucose tolerance in children and adolescents. J Diabetes. 2015;7 (1):10-5.

5

The Effect of Ergogenic Supplements and Mediterranean Diet on Cycling Performance; Differences According to Duration and Intensity

Sousana Papadopoulou[1], Elpiniki Kroustalloudi[1], Ioannis Pagkalos[1,2], Anna Kokkinopoulou[1], and Maria Hassapidou[1]

[1]Department of Nutrition & Dietetics, Alexander Technological Educational Institute of Thessaloniki, Sindos, Thessaloniki, Greece
[2]Department of Electrical & Computer Engineering, Aristotle University of Thessaloniki, Thessaloniki, Greece

Corresponding Author: Maria Hassapidou; email: mnhas@nutr.teithe.gr

Abstract

Aims: To record the prevalence and the type of supplement use among cyclists and to estimate the effect of caffeine, carbohydrates, energy drinks and meddiet score on 200m and 4km cycling time-trial performances in a Greek sample. **Methods:** Fifty male cycling athletes aged 32 ± 20 years participated in a randomized, double-blind study. The subjects were submitted to anthropometric measurements and body composition was assessed with bioelectrical impedance. All participants completed the meddiet Score questionnaire and a validated questionnaire about their ergogenic aids' preference. The athletes performed two cycling trials (200m and 4km) and their records were taken down and were evaluated according to their consumption of caffeine, carbohydrates and energy drinks and their meddiet score. For the statistical analysis SPSS, v20 was used. **Results:** Greek cyclists had a mean BMI value of 23.65 ± 2.74 and a mean body fat percentage of 15.82 ± 8.33. Endurance and speed performances were improved with caffeine consumption when compared to no consumption (7.42 ± 3.92 min vs 12.5 ± 3.16 min, $p < 0.001$ and 20.75 ± 15.69 sec vs 34.07 ± 16.25 sec, $p < 0.05$, respectively), as well as with energy drinks' consumption (8.77 ± 4.15 min vs 13.25 ± 2.47 min, $p < 0.001$ and 20.35 ± 14.08 sec vs 39.14±14.38 sec, $p<0.001$, respectively). Carbohydrates' intake improved performance in the endurance test (7.60 ± 3.72 min vs 12.86 ± 2.92 min, $p < 0.001$), but did not have a positive influence in the speed test (25.73 ± 18.68 sec vs 33.08 ± 15.95 sec, $p > 0.05$). **Conclusions:** Ergogenic aids had a positive effect on the athletic performance in terms of speed and endurance in cyclists.

Keywords: Cycling, Athletic performance, Ergogenic aids, Mediterranean diet

1. Introduction

Dietary supplement use is expanding among athletes who are experimenting with a variety of substances, even illegal ones as to reach a competitive edge [15, 25, 33]. Ranges of age of cyclists vary and some athletes remain highly competitive into their 40s, although it is likely that performance peaks before 35 years of age. Ageing performance declines in similar way among several sports, yet, there are older, competitive and athletically ambitious athletes, called veterans or masters. Most likely to be founded positive for illegal substances are non-professional cyclists aged 30 to 50 years. Therefore, cycling is one of the most energy-expensive sports and the use of ergogenic aids is most popular [33].

Maintaining performance during endurance exercise is dependent on a variety of dietary factors, such as energy and water balance, appropriate macro and micronutrient intake. [19]. Many athletes do not seem to cover their energy demands [27] and are often leaded to limited energy supply [45, 55, 59, 82].

The main nutrient that can improve endurance and reduce fatigue is carbohydrates [20, 72], through maintaining blood glucose levels, CHO oxidation rates and preventing glycogen depletion [13]. Athletes consuming high proportion of carbohydrates had a better performance compared to others who consumed moderate quantities [14, 16, 38]. However, carbohydrates' consumption before and during brief exercise cannot act favorably [13].

Thus, carbohydrates act as ergogenic aid in endurance sports as cycling [13]. Other preferred ergogenic aids of cyclists, except for carbohydrates, are: proteins, caffeine, creatine, sodium bicarbonate beta-alanine and nitrates [18].

Sport beverages gained popularity as they attribute to both energy-giving and hydration- and electrolyte status maintaining in endurance performance. Experienced and older athletes are more likely to prefer sport beverages and to follow a drinking schedule during exercise [58, 88]. Energy drinks seem, also, to have a positive effect on performance [78] through hydration and energy supply [24, 37] and fatigue reduction [2, 14] and thus, they are of vital importance for endurance sports [39]. Elements contained in energy drinks are ginseng, guarana, taurine and caffeine which are not dangerous when received in recommended doses [17].

Caffeine can improve performance [7, 79] acting through an enhance in central nervous system and in fat oxidation rate [68, 86]. There are many studies suggesting that caffeine improves power and endurance compared to placebo or other supplements [26, 29, 35, 54, 57, 81]. A moderate dose of caffeine significantly improves performance

[44, 84], while very low doses of caffeine cannot be ergogenic [6] and a high dose may act against performance [48]. Chronic ingestion of low caffeine doses develops tolerance in low-caffeine consumers. Therefore, individuals with low-habitual intakes should refrain from chronic caffeine supplementation as to maximize performance benefits from acute caffeine ingestion [6].

American Dietetic Association, Dietitians of Canada and the American College of Sports state that anthropometric characteristics influence performance. Body composition and weight are the two main factors that can be manipulated and contribute to potential for athletic success. Specifically, body weight can add to an athlete's endurance, speed and power, while body composition improves agility, strength and appearance. However body mass and composition cannot solely predict the progression of a career and there is no optimal competitive body weight or composition for any sport or athletic group [74, 86]. Thus, body weight and composition are important indicators of physical fitness and can improve performance [3, 42]. Low body fat and high muscle mass levels are linked with better sports achievements [42].

Mediterranean diet contains an abundance of bioactive food constituents like complex carbohydrates, fibers, vegetable proteins, unsaturated fas, minerals, vitamins, polyphenols and phytosterols that can interact synergistically and affect beneficially metabolic pathways, lowering the risk of cardiometabolic disorders, cognitive decline and all-cause mortality [47, 75, 80]. Endurance exercise generates oxidative stress and acute inflammation [12], whereas Mediterranean diet improves immune system function [50], mitigates inflammation and enhances performance, recovery and injury repair [76]. For these reasons adherence to Mediterranean diet is essential for athletes following an exhaustive training program such as cyclists. Meddiet score is a useful tool that can evaluate the adherence to Mediterranean dietary pattern [60].

There is limited data regarging nutrition practices and energy needs of elite athletes, especially in Greece [31, 32, 61, 63, 64, 66, 67]. To the best of our knowledge there is no study on the effect of ergogenic aids and meddiet score on Greek cyclists' performance. Therefore, the goals of the present study were to record the prevalence and the type of supplement use among cyclists and to estimate the effect of caffeine, carbohydrates, energy drinks and meddiet score on 200m and 4km cycling time-trial performance in a Greek sample.

2. Methods

2.1. Population Sample

Fifty male cyclists aged 32 ± 20 years participated in this randomized double-blind study. Athletes responded to an announcement for this study posted in different cycling local training teams. Fifty cyclists fulfilled the inclusion criteria of the study (having a background for at least 6 sequentially years of training, having competed in the Greek National Championship and not having any orthopaedic/neuromuscular, restraining problems or taking any steroid supplements). The study was carried out in Thessaloniki, Greece, in 2015.

Participants have given their written consent prior to entering the study, which received approval by the Ethics Committee of the Alexander Technological Educational Institute of Thessaloniki, Greece, and is in accordance with the Declaration of Helsinki.

2.2. Procedures

The present study was divided into three meetings.

2.2.1. Anthropometric Characteristics and Body Composition

The first meeting took place one day before the first cycling trial. In the first meeting, an experienced dietitian performed all anthropometric measurements in the morning, after an overnight fasting and all athletes were in minimal clothing. Body weight was measured with the use of a calibrated digital scale with an accuracy of ±100g (Tanita 545N) and body height to the nearest 0.5 cm using a stadiometer, with an accuracy of 0.5 cm (SECA 220). Body mass index (BMI) was calculated as body weight divided by the square of height (kg/m^2). Body composition was estimated with the method of bioelectrical impedance analysis using portable bioelectrical impedance device (Tanita 545N). All cyclists were informed about the protocol for body composition assessment. They abstained from any type of exercise one day prior to measurement. Cyclists stood bare feet on the device, maintaining contact with their feet on electrodes and instructed to grasp the retractable handle as to have contact on electrodes with their palms.

2.2.2. Questionnaires

During the first meeting, a qualified dietitian instructed all subjects to complete the meddiet Score [60] and a questionnaire that has been evaluated in a previous study

Anthropometric characteristics	Min	Max	Mean	SD
Weight (kg)	51.00	123.00	74.6	12.2
Height (m)	1.61	1.92	1.77	0.08
Body Fat (%)	5.80	36.40	15.82	8.33
Body Water (%)	50.20	69.10	58.51	4.15
BMI (kg/m2)	19.00	33.40	23.65	2.74

TABLE 1: Anthropometric characteristics.

from our lab, regarding their ergogenic supplements' consumption (ie. Type of supplement, reasons for their use, source of information) [62, 65].

2.2.3. Cycling Trials

In the second meeting, all athletes completed a field based 200m speed race. In the third meeting, they completed a field based 4km endurance race. Their performance was evaluated according to the ergogenic supplement that each athlete had received, and their meddiet score.

2.3. Statistical Analysis

For the statistical analysis and the elaboration of the results, the computer package SPSS v20 was used. Results are presented as means ± standard deviation and/or percentages where appropriate. The level of significance was set at $p<0.05$.

3. Results

A total of 50 male cyclists participated in the study, with their age varying from 15 to 50 years.

Table 1 depicts anthropometric characteristics of our sample.

Frequency of training is presented in table 2. Each session lasted 1.5h, approximately.

Cyclists used 10 different nutritional supplements (Table 3). 44% of the cyclists consumed energy drinks, while caffeine, carbohydrates, proteins and vitamins were used by 24%, 30%, 30% and 22%, respectively. Also, it is worth to mention that 38% of the athletes did not take any supplement in order to improve their performance.

Sessions per week	N	Percentage
1-3 / week	13	26%
3-6 / week	24	47%
6-7 / week	14	27%

TABLE 2: Frequency of training.

Ergogenic aids	N	Percentage
Energy drinks	22	44%
Athletic drinks	9	18%
Caffeine	12	24%
Carbohydrates	15	30%
Protein / Acids	15	30%
Sodium	1	2%
Vitamins / Minerals	11	22%
Creatine	2	4%
Carnitine	3	6%
Glutamine	4	8%
Nothing	19	38%

TABLE 3: Supplements consumption.

Endurance and speed performances were improved with caffeine consumption when compared to no consumption (7.42 ± 3.92 min vs 12.5 ± 3.16 min, $p < 0.001$ and 20.75 ± 15.69 sec vs 34.07 ± 16.25 sec, $p < 0.05$, respectively), as well as with energy drinks' consumption (8.77 ± 4.15 min vs 13.25 ± 2.47 min, $p < 0.001$ and 20.35 ± 14.08 sec vs 39.14 ± 14.38 sec, $p < 0.001$, respectively). Carbohydrates' intake improved performance in the endurance test (7.60 ± 3.72 min vs 12.86 ± 2.92 min, $p < 0.001$), but did not have a positive influence in the speed test (25.73 ± 18.68 sec vs 33.08 ± 15.95 sec, $p > 0.05$) (Table 4).

Adherence to the Mediterranean diet was assessed by the meddiet Score (theoretical range: 0-55). Forty-three out of 50 cyclists had a median score regarding the adherence to the Mediterranean diet (score 28-41), while six cyclists had low scores (score 14-27) and only 1 cyclist had great adherence to the Mediterranean diet. Level of adherence to the Mediterranean diet played no significant role in endurance ($p = 0.563$) and speed test results ($p = 0.462$) (Table 5).

Supplements' consumption		N	Endurance performance (minutes)	Speed Performance (seconds)
	Yes	12	7.42 ± 3.92 (p = 0.001)	20.75 ± 15.69 (p = 0.016)
Caffeine	No	38	12.5 ± 3.16 (p = 0.001)	34.07 ± 16.25 (p = 0.016)
	Yes	15	7.60 ± 3.72 (p = 0.001)	25.73 ± 18.68 (p = 0.163)
Carbohydrates	No	35	12.86 ± 2.92 (p = 0.001)	33.08 ± 15.95 (p = 0.163)
	Yes	22	8.77 ± 4.15 (p = 0.001)	20.35 ± 14.08 (p = 0.001)
Energy drinks	No	28	13.25 ± 2.47 (p = 0.001)	39.14 ± 14.38 (p = 0.001)
Total cyclists regardless supplement consumption		50	11.28 ± 3.97 (p = 0.001)	30.88 ± 16.96 (p = 0.001)

TABLE 4: Performance in endurance and speed tests according to supplements' consumption.

Meddiet Score	N	Performance of resistance (minutes)	Performance of speed (seconds)
Score 14-27	6	12.50 ± 3.56 (p = 0.563)	30.63 ± 18.63 (p = 0.462)
Score 28-41	43	11.05 ± 4.06 (p = 0.563)	30.42 ± 16.84 (p = 0.462)
Score 42-55	1	14.00 (p = 0.563)	32.00 (p = 0.462)

TABLE 5: Performance in endurance and speed tests according to adherence to the Mediterranean diet.

4. Discussion

As it regards, the anthropometric variables, Greek cyclists had a mean BMI value of 23.65 ± 2.74 and a mean body fat percentage of 15.82 ± 8.33. Cyclists of the present study had higher values in both BMI and body fat levels compared to 6 professional road cyclists participated in the Tour of Andalusia, a 4stage race covering 647.6 Km [77]. In comparison to other endurance sports, Greek cyclists presented similar BMI and body fat levels with Greek male cross country skiers [63], with the New Zealand Ironman triathlon male athletes [41] and with the non-professional male triathletes, that participated in the Daurada Extreme Man Salou-Costa triathlon [4].

According to [42], high body fat affects negatively cyclists' performance and increased BMI acts against racing effort [5, 40]. In [85] investigated the effects of training and anthropometric characteristics on male marathon and ultra-marathon performance and found that body fat levels above 15% can negatively affect performance.

In our sample, most cyclists trained less than 9 hours per week, which is less than the appropriate training load that maximizes athletes' performance, according to [73].

In the present study, 62% of the cyclists took supplements in order to improve their performance. A total of 44% of the cyclists consumed energy drinks, while caffeine, carbohydrates and proteins and vitamins were used by 24% 30%, 30% and 22%, respectively. A small percentage of Greek cyclists consumed carnitine, which lacks scientific evidence for boosting performance [10, 86].

A recent study of [87] in 778 Dutch athletes with elite status, reported that when athletes received dietary counseling had a higher consumption of vitamin D, isotonic drinks, recovery drinks, energy bars, isotonic sports drinks with protein, probiotics, beta-alanine and sodium bicarbonate. In contrast when they did not have any counseling, they preferred combined vitamin supplements, calcium, energy gels BCAA/ other amino acids and energy drinks.

Previous studies reported that dietary supplements are used by athletes as to allow them to improve performance through harder training, quicker recover (Ziegler et al., 2003), [52] and prevention from injuries and illness (Ziegler et al., 2003), [69]. The prevalence of dietary supplementation among elite athletes falls in the range of 62–91% for athletes under 20 years of age [9, 22, 23, 56], and 51–99% for elite adult athletes [9, 21, 23, 36, 83, 87].

The use of dietary supplements is alarming as athletes consume different supplements [21, 22, 69] that can interact with each other [10, 71] or provoke negative consequences such as allergic reactions or toxicity in large doses (Lawson et al., 2007), [71] or have as a result misinformation [49] and inadvertent product contamination [28]. There is lack in universal regulation and consequently there are differences across countries in the ergogenic aids' practice and approach. There is often a gap between scientific evidence and marketing hype [71].

Regarding the impact of supplementation on cycling performance, the present study concluded that energy drinks' consumption was associated with better performance in both endurance ($p = 0.001$) and speed races ($p = 0.001$), a finding which comes in agreement with other studies in cyclists showing that performance was improved with energy drinks comparing to placebo [1, 24, 37]. We should bare in mind that energy drinks should be consumed in rational proportions as to act in favor of exercise, otherwise they may become dangerous, causing hypertension, cardiac dysrhythmias, tachycardia or heart failure [17, 24, 71].

Accordingly, in the present study, carbohydrates showed a positive impact on athletic performance during the endurance test ($p = 0.001$), similar with other experimental studies in cyclists [20, 46]. However, regarding the speed test of 200m, the consumption of carbohydrates from our cyclists did not have any ergogenic benefit ($p = 0.163$), which is suggested by [13].

Finally, our results indicated that caffeine consumption improved performance in both endurance and speed races, when comparing to other cyclists who did not consume caffeine. The ergogenic impact of caffeine is supported by a plethora of studies [8, 26, 30, 34, 35]. However, caffeine intake can provoke side effects such as headache, hypertension, tachycardia and gastrointestinal upset [11, 51] and acts differently in every athlete [70].

Regarding the results from the meddiet Score, 86% of our cyclists had a median adherence to the Mediterranean diet, whereas 12% had a low adherence. This finding is in accordance with a study in 45 young Spanish cyclists, reporting that approximately 20% of them did not comply to the Mediterranean diet, confirming a gradual abandoning of the Mediterranean Diet [76].

In the present study, there was no significant effect of the Mediterranean diet on speed or endurance cycling performance. To the best of our knowledge there is no study estimating the effect of Mediterranean diet on sport performance.

5. Conclusion

The current study provides insight into supplement use of Greek cyclists. The consumption of carbohydrates, caffeine and energy drinks was beneficial for the cycling performance. Athletes lack knowledge about ergogenic aids, as they are often consulted by their coaches who had limited nutrition and ergogenic aids information. The presence of certified sports dietitians is vital in order to maximize athletes' records and protect them from receiving useless aids.

Further research is needed to evaluate supplement use of athletes, in combination with their nutrition status and Mediterranean diet adherence in larger groups of athletes. Variables, like duration of supplementation, quantity and type of supplements should be considered in future studies as they might have beneficial or adverse effects on cyclists' performance. Given the widespread use of supplements, dietitians and physicians have to collaborate in order to counsel cyclists about supplements' effectiveness, safety and legality.

6. Limitations

The results regarding the impact of ergogenic aids such as caffeine, carbohydrates and energy drinks on cycling performance should be presented with reservation, as the sample was small and we did not take into account the quantity, frequency and combined use of ergogenic supplements received by each athlete.

References

[1] Abian P, Del Coso J, Salinero JJ, Gallo-Salazar C, Areces F, Ruiz-Vicente D, Lara B, Soriano L, Muñoz V, Abian-Vicen J. The ingestion of a caffeinated energy drink improves jump performance and activity patterns in elite badminton players. J Sports Sci. 2015; 33: 1042–1050.

[2] Anastasiou CA, Kavouras SA, Koutsari C, Georgakakis C, Skenderi K, Beer M, Sidossis LS. Effect of maltose-containing sports drinks on exercise performance. Int J Sport Nutr Exerc Metab. 2004; 14: 609–625.

[3] Arrese AL, Ostáriz ES. Skinfold thicknesses associated with distance running performance in highly trained runners. J Sports Sci. 2006; 24: 69–76.

[4] Barrero A, Erola P, Bescós R. Energy balance of triathletes during an ultra-endurance event. Nutrients. 2014; 7(1): 209-222.

[5] Beattie K, Carson BP, Lyons M, Kenny IC. The Effect of Maximal- & Explosive-Strength Training on Performance Indicators in Cyclists. Int J Sports Physiol Perform. 2016; 1–25.

[6] Beaumont R, Cordery P, Funnell M, Mears S, James L, Watson P. Chronic ingestion of a low dose of caffeine induces tolerance to the performance benefits of caffeine. J Sports Sci. 2016; 1–8.

[7] Black CD, Waddell DE, Gonglach AR. Caffeine's Ergogenic Effects on Cycling: Neuromuscular and Perceptual Factors. Med Sci Sports Exerc. 2015; 47: 1145–1158.

[8] Bortolotti H, Altimari LR, Vitor-Costa M, Cyrino ES. Performance during a 20-km cycling time-trial after caffeine ingestion. J Int Soc Sports Nutr. 2014; 11: 45.

[9] Braun H, Koehler K, Geyer H, Kleinert J, Mester J, Schänzer W. Dietary supplement use among elite young German athletes. Int J Sport Nutr Exer Metab. 2009; 19(1): 97-109.

[10] Broad EM, Maughan RJ, Galloway SDR. Effects of four weeks L-carnitine L-tartrate ingestion on substrate utilization during prolonged exercise. Int J Sport Nutr Exerc Metab. 2005; 15: 665–679.

[11] Brooks JH, Wyld K, Chrismas BC. Caffeine Supplementation as an Ergogenic Aid for Muscular Strength and Endurance: A Recommendation for Coaches and Athletes. J Athl Enhanc. 2016.

[12] Brunngard H. Physical activity and modulation of systemic low-level inflammation. J Leukoc Biol 2005; 78(4): 819-835.

[13] Burke LM, Hawley JA, Wong SH, Jeukendrup AE. Carbohydrates for training and competition. J Sports Sci. 2011; 29(Suppl 1): S17-S27.

[14] Burke LM, Millet G, Tarnopolsky MA. International Association of Athletics Federations, Nutrition for distance events. J Sports Sci. 2007; 25(Suppl 1): S29-38.

[15] Calfee R, Fadale P. Popular Ergogenic Drugs and Supplements in Young Athletes. Pediatrics. 2006; 117: 577–589.

[16] Chlíbková D, Knechtle B, Rosemann T, Tomášková I, Chadim V, Shortall M. Nutrition habits in 24-hour mountain bike racers. Springer Plus. 2014; 3: 715.

[17] Clauson KA, Shields KM, mcqueen CE, Persad N. Safety issues associated with commercially available energy drinks. J Am Pharm Assoc. 2008; 48: 55-67

[18] Close GL, Hamilton DL, Philp A, Burke LM, Morton JP. New strategies in sport nutrition to increase exercise performance. Free Radic Biol Med. 2016; 98: 144–158.

[19] Colombani PC, Mannhart C, Wenk C, Frey WO. Nutritional intake during a 244 km multisport ultraendurance race. Pakistan Journal of Nutrition. 2002; 1(3): 124-126.

[20] Correia-Oliveira CR, Bertuzzi R, Dal'Molin Kiss MAP, Lima-Silva A.E. Strategies of dietary carbohydrate manipulation and their effects on performance in cycling time trials. Sports Med Auckl NZ. 2013; 43: 707–719.

[21] Dascombe BJ, Karunaratna M, Cartoon J, Fergie B, Goodman C. Nutritional supplementation habits and perceptions of elite athletes within a state-based sporting institute. J Sci Med Sport. 2010; 13(2): 274–280.

[22] Diehl K, Thiel A, Zipfel S, Mayer J, Schnell A, Schneider S. Elite Adolescent Athletes' Use of Dietary Supplements: Characteristics, Opinions, and Sources of Supply and Information. Int J Sport Nutr Exer Metab. 2012; 22: 165 -174.

[23] Erdman KA, Fung TS, Doyle-Baker PK, Verhoef MJ, Reimer RA. Dietary supplementation of high-performance Canadian athletes by age and gender. Clin J Sport Med. 2007; 17(6): 458-464.

[24] Eudy AE, Gordon LL, Hockaday BC, Lee DA, Lee V, Luu D, Martinez CA, Ambrose PJ. Efficacy and safety of ingredients found in preworkout supplements. Am J Health-Syst Pharm. 2013; 70: 577–588.

[25] Foddy B, Savulescu J. Ethics of performance enhancement in sport: drugs and gene doping. Principles of Health Care Ethics, Second Edition. 2007; 511-519.

[26] Ganio MS, Klau JF, Casa DJ, Armstrong LE, Maresh CM. Effect of caffeine on sport-specific endurance performance: a systematic review. J Strength Cond Res. 2009; 23: 315–324.

[27] Geesmann B, Mester J, Koehler K. Energy balance, macronutrient intake, and hydration status during a 1,230 km ultra-endurance bike marathon. Int J Sport Nutr Exerc Metab. 2014; 24: 497–506.

[28] Geyer H, Parr MK, Koehler K, Mareck U, Schδnzer W, Thevis M. Nutritional supplements crosscontaminated and faked with doping substances. Journal of Mass Spectrometry. 2008; 43(7): 892–902.

[29] Glaister M, Pattison JR, Muniz-Pumares D, Patterson SD, Foley P. Effects of dietary nitrate, caffeine, and their combination on 20-km cycling time trial performance. J Strength Cond Res. 2015; 29: 165–174.

[30] Graham-Paulson T, Perret C, Goosey-Tolfrey V. Improvements in Cycling but Not Handcycling 10 km Time Trial Performance in Habitual Caffeine Users. Nutrients. 2016; 8(7): 393.

[31] Hassapidou NM, Manstrantoni A. Dietary intakes of elite female athletes in Greece. J Hum Nutr Diet. 2001; 14: 391-396.

[32] Hassapidou MN, Fourtounopoulos D, Efstratiou E, Kitsou S, Papakitsos C. Dietary intakes of Greek basketball players. Nutr Food Sci. 2003; 33(1): 23-27.

[33] Henning AD, Dimeo P. The complexities of anti-doping violations: a case study of sanctioned cases in all performance levels of USA cycling. Perform Enhanc Health. 2014; 3: 159–166.

[34] Higgins S, Straight CR, Lewis RD. The Effects of Preexercise Caffeinated Coffee Ingestion on Endurance Performance: An Evidence-Based Review. Int J Sport Nutr Exerc Metab. 2016; 26: 221–239.

[35] Hodgson AB, Randell RK, Jeukendrup AE. The metabolic and performance effects of caffeine compared to coffee during endurance exercise. Plos One. 2013; 8(4): 59561.

[36] Huang SHS, Johnson K, Pipe AL. The use of dietary supplements and medications by Canadian athletes at the Atlanta and Sydney Olympic Games. Clin J Sport Med. 2006; 16(1): 27-33.

[37] Ivy JL, Kammer L, Ding Z, Wang B, Bernard JR, Liao Y-H, Hwang J. Improved cycling time-trial performance after ingestion of a caffeine energy drink. Int J Sport Nutr Exerc Metab. 2009; 19: 61–78.

[38] Jeukendrup AE, Hopkins S, Aragón-Vargas LF, Hulston C. No effect of carbohydrate feeding on 16 km cycling time trial performance. Eur J Appl Physiol. 2008; 104: 831–837.

[39] Khanna, GL, Manna I. Supplementary effect of carbohydrate-electrolyte drink on sports performance, lactate removal & cardiovascular response of athletes. Indian J Med Res. 2005; 121: 665–669.

[40] Khodaee M, Olewinski L, Shadgan B, Kiningham RR. Rapid Weight Loss in Sports with Weight Classes. Curr Sports Med Rep. 2015; 14: 435–441.

[41] Kimber NE, Ross JJ, Mason SL. Speedy DB. (2002). Energy balance during an ironman triathlon in male and female triathletes. Int J Sport Nutr Exerc Metab. 2012; 12: 47-62.

[42] Knechtle B, Wirth A, Rüst CA, Rosemann T. The Relationship between Anthropometry and Split Performance in Recreational Male Ironman Triathletes. Asian J Sports Med. 2011; 2: 23–30.

[43] Knechtle B, Zingg MA, Rosemann T, Stiefel M, Rüst CA. What predicts performance in ultra-triathlon races? - a comparison between Ironman distance triathlon and ultra-triathlon. Open Access J Sports Med. 2015; 6: 149–159.

[44] Lane SC, Areta JL, Bird SR, Coffey VG, Burke LM, Desbrow B, Karagounis LG, Hawley JA. Caffeine ingestion and cycling power output in a low or normal muscle glycogen state. Med Sci Sports Exerc. 2013; 45: 1577–1584.

[45] Lee MJC, Hammond KM, Vasdev A, Poole KL, Impey SG, Close GL, Morton JP. Self-selecting fluid intake while maintaining high carbohydrate availability does not impair half-marathon performance. Int J Sports Med. 2014; 35: 1216–1222.

[46] Little JP, Chilibeck PD, Ciona D, Forbes S, Rees H, Vandenberg A, Zello GA. Effect of low- and high-glycemic-index meals on metabolism and performance during high-intensity, intermittent exercise. Int J Sport Nutr Exerc Metab. 2010; 20: 447–456.

[47] Lourida I, Soni M, Thompson-Coon J, Purandare N, Lang IA, Ukoumunne OC, Llewellyn DJ. Mediterranean diet, cognitive function, and dementia: a systematic review. Epidemiology. 2013; 24(4): 479-489.

[48] Lystrup RM, Leggit JC. Caffeine Toxicity Due to Supplement Use in Caffeine-Naïve Individual: A Cautionary Tale. Mil Med. 2015; 180: 936-940.

[49] Malinauskas BM, Overton RF, Carraway VG, Cash BC. Supplements of interest for sport-related injury and sources of supplement information among college athletes. Advances in Medical Sciences. 2007; 52: 50–54.

[50] Marcos A, Nova E, Montero A. Changes in the immune system are conditioned by nutrition. Eur J Clin Nutr. 2003; 57(1): S66-S69.

[51] Martínez-Sellés M, Datino T, Figueiras-Graillet L, Gama JG, Jones C, Franklin R, Fernández-Avilés F. Cardiovascular Safety of Anagrelide in Healthy Subjects: Effects of Caffeine and Food Intake on Pharmacokinetics and Adverse Reactions. Clin Drug Investig. 2013; 33: 45–54.

[52] Maughan RJ, King DS, Lea T. Dietary supplements. J Sports Sci. 2004; 22(1): 95–113.

[53] Maughan RJ. 2005. Contamination of dietary supplements and positive drug tests in sport. J Sports Sci. 2005; 23(9): 883–889.

[54] Miller B, O'Connor H, Orr R, Ruell P, Cheng HL, Chow CM. Combined caffeine and carbohydrate ingestion: effects on nocturnal sleep and exercise performance in athletes. Eur J Appl Physiol. 2014; 114: 2529–2537.

[55] Nicolò A, Bazzucchi I, Felici F, Patrizio F, Sacchetti M. Mechanical and electromyographic responses during the 3-min all-out test in competitive cyclists. J Electromyogr Kinesiol. 2015; 25: 907–913.

[56] Nieper A. Nutritional supplement practices in UK junior national track and field athletes. Br J Sports Med. 2015; 39(9): 645-649.

[57] Nikolopoulos DD, Spiliopoulou C, Theocharis SE. Doping and musculoskeletal system: short-term and long-lasting effects of doping agents. Fundam Clin Pharmacol. 2011; 25: 535–563.

[58] O'Neal EK, Wingo JE, Richardson MT, Leeper JD, Neggers YH, Bishop PA. Half-marathon and full-marathon runners' hydration practices and perceptions. J Athl Train. 2011; 46(6): 581-591.

[59] Ormsbee MJ, Bach CW, Baur DA. Pre-Exercise Nutrition: The Role of Macronutrients, Modified Starches and Supplements on Metabolism and Endurance Performance. Nutrients. 2014; 6: 1782–1808.

[60] Panagiotakos DB, Pitsavos C, Stefanadis C. Dietary patterns: a Mediterranean diet score and its relation to clinical and biological markers of cardiovascular disease risk. Nutr Metab Cardiovasc Dis. 2006; 16(8): 559-568.

[61] Papandreou D, Eystathiadis P, Bouzoukiu V, Hassapidou M, Tsitskaris G, Garefis A. Dietary assessment, anthropometric measurements and nutritional status of Greek professional athletes. Nutr Food Sci. 2007; 37(5): 338-344.

[62] Papadopoulou SK. Food Choice criteria of adolescents. The role of physical activity and anthropometric, dietetic and psychological factors. Unpublished Dissertation, Aristotle University of Thessaloniki, Greece. 2001.

[63] Papadopoulou SK, Gouvianaki A, Grammatikopoulou MG, Maraki Z, Pangalos IG, Hassapidou MN. Body fat status and energy and nutrient intake of elite cross-country skiers, members of the Greek national team. Asian J Sports Med. 2012; 3(4): 257-266.

[64] Papadopoulou SK, Papadopoulou SD. Nutritional status of team sport athletes according to body fat status. Nutr Food Sci. 2010; 40:64-73.

[65] Papadopoulou SD, Papadopoulou SK, Zaggelidis G, Konstantinidou X, Tsitskaris G, Maraki Z. Dietary and health related habits of Greek elite female team sport athletes. Stiinta Sportului "Sports Science magazine". 2009; 1: 79-91.

[66] Papadopoulou SK, Papadopoulou SD, Skoufas D, Yiannakos A, Natsis K. Dietary intake differences between volleyball and handball women athletes of the Olympic national team. Medicina Sportiva. 2008; 16: 983-989.

[67] Papadopoulou SK, Papadopoulou SD, Gallos GK. Macro and Micro-nutrient Intake of Adolescent Greek Female Volleyball players. Int J Sport Nutr Exerc Metab. 2002; 12: 73-80.

[68] Paton C, Costa V, Guglielmo L. Effects of caffeine chewing gum on race performance and physiology in male and female cyclists. J Sports Sci. 2015; 33: 1076–1083.

[69] Petróczi A, Naughton DP, Pearce G, Bailey R, Bloodworth A, mcnamee M. Nutritional supplement use by elite young UK athletes: Fallacies of advice regarding efficacy. J Int Soc Sport Nutr. 2008; 5: 22.

[70] Pettitt RW, Niemeyer JD, Sexton PJ, Lipetzky A, Murray SR. Do the noncaffeine ingredients of energy drinks affect metabolic responses to heavy exercise? J Strength Cond Res. 2013; 27: 1994–1999.

[71] Porrini M, Del Bo' C. Ergogenic Aids and Supplements. In Sports Endocrinology (Vol. 47, pp. 128-152). Karger Publishers. 2016.

[72] Pöchmüller M, Schwingshackl L, Colombani PC, Hoffmann G. A systematic review and meta-analysis of carbohydrate benefits associated with randomized controlled competition-based performance trials. J Int Soc Sports Nutr. 2016; 13(1): 27.

[73] Quiterio AL, Carnero EA, Silva AM, Baptista F, Sardinha LB. Weekly training hours are associated with molecular and cellular body composition levels in adolescent athletes. J Sports Med Phys Fitness. 2009; 49: 54–63.

[74] Rodriguez NR, dimarco NM, Langley S, American Dietetic Association, Dietitians of Canada, American College of Sports Medicine: Nutrition and Athletic Performance. Position of the American Dietetic Association, Dietitians of Canada, and the American College of Sports Medicine: Nutrition and athletic performance. J Am Diet Assoc. 2009; 109: 509–527.

[75] Salas-Salvadó J, Guasch-Ferré M, Lee CH, Estruch R, Clish CB, Ros E. Protective effects of the Mediterranean diet on type 2 diabetes and metabolic syndrome. J Nutr. 2016; 146(4): S920- S927.

[76] Sánchez-Benito JL, Sánchez-Soriano E, Ginart Suárez J. Assessment of the Mediterranean Diet Adequacy Index of a collective of young cyclists. Nutr Hosp. 2009; 24: 77–86.

[77] Sánchez-Muñoz C, Zabala M, Muros JJ. Nutritional intake and anthropometric changes of professional road cyclists during a 4-day competition. Scand J Med Sci Sports. 2016; 26: 802–808.

[78] Shearer J, Graham TE. Performance effects and metabolic consequences of caffeine and caffeinated energy drink consumption on glucose disposal. Nutr Rev. 2014; 72(Suppl 1): 121–136.

[79] Siegel-Tike P, Rosales-Soto G, Herrera Valenzuela T, Durán Agüero S, Yáñez Sepúlveda R. Body composition parameters and relationship with the maximal aerobic power in recreational cyclists. Nutr Hosp. 2015; 32: 2223–2227.

[80] Sofi F, Abbate R, Gensini GF, Casini A. Accruing evidence on benefits of adherence to the Mediterranean diet on health: an updated systematic review and meta-analysis. Am J Clin Nutr. 2010; 92: 1189–1196.

[81] Spence AL, Sim M, Landers G, Peeling P. A comparison of caffeine versus pseudoephedrine on cycling time-trial performance. Int J Sport Nutr Exerc Metab. 2013; 23: 507–512.

[82] Stellingwerff T, Maughan RJ, Burke LM. Nutrition for power sports: middle-distance running, track cycling, rowing, canoeing/kayaking, and swimming. J Sports Sci. 2011; 29(Suppl 1): S79-89.

[83] Suzic Lazic J, Dikic N, Radivojevic N, Mazic S, Radovanovic D, Mitrovic N, Lazic M, Zivanic S, Suzic S. Dietary supplements and medications in elite sport–polypharmacy or real need? Scand J Med Sci Sports. 2011; 21(2): 260-267.

[84] Talanian JL, Spriet LL. Low and moderate doses of caffeine late in exercise improve performance in trained cyclists. Appl Physiol Nutr Metab. 2016; 41: 850–855.

[85] Tanda G, Knechtle B. Effects of training and anthropometric factors on marathon and 100 km ultramarathon race performance. Open Access J Sports Med. 2015; 6: 129–136.

[86] Thomas DT, Erdman KA, Burke LM. Position of the Academy of Nutrition and Dietetics, Dietitians of Canada, and the American College of Sports Medicine: Nutrition and Athletic Performance. J Acad Nutr Diet. 2016; 116: 501–528.

[87] Wardenaar FC, Ceelen IJ, Van Dijk JW, Hangelbroek RW, Van Roy L, Van der Pouw B, De Vries JHM, Mensink M. Witkamp RF. Nutritional Supplement Use by Dutch Elite and Sub-Elite Athletes: Does Receiving Dietary Counselling Make a Difference? Int J Sport Nutr Exerc Metab. 2016; 1-25.

[88] Winger JM, Dugas JP, Dugas LR. Beliefs about hydration and physiology drive drinking behaviours in runners. Br J Sports Med. 2011; 45(8): 646-649.

6

The Effect of Breakfast on Academic Performance among High School Students in Abu Dhabi

Zainab Taha and Ayesha S. Rashed

College of Narural and Health Sciences, Zayed University, Abu Dhabi, U.A.E

Corresponding Author: Zainab Taha; email: zainab.taha@zu.ac.ae

Abstract

Background: The claim that breakfast is the most important meal of the day has an abundance of sound science behind it. Breakfast is continually suggested to be a critical feature of eating regimens since it is associated with a healthier intake of nutrients, BMI and lifestyle. Several studies have shown the importance of having breakfast to the body's performance. Moreover, recent studies have demonstrated that breakfast enhances intellectual capacity, concentration, attention and academic performance. However, there is a paucity of studies which examine the relationship between breakfast consumption and academic performance in the UAE. **Objective:** The aim of this study is to examine the effect of breakfast intake on the academic performance of young female students in the emirate of Abu Dhabi. **Methods:** Data was collected through a self-administered questionnaire from 130 female students aged 15-19 years, who were selected from two private schools in Abu Dhabi. The questionnaire was used to explore the students' breakfast consumption habits. The data collected was analyzed to examine the association between breakfast intake and academic performance. Academic performance was assessed according to the average grade for all subjects in the final exam. **Results:** Sixty-two percent of the 130 students eat breakfast regularly. Breakfast consumption is associated with increased academic performance among high school female students. The association of breakfast intake was found to be statistically significant ($p = 0.00$). **Conclusion:** The findings of the current study indicate that there is a positive correlation between breakfast intake and the students' scores. Regular breakfast consumption improves students' academic performance, whereas the performance of students who frequently skip breakfast is lower.

Keywords: Breakfast, Students, Academic performance, Abu Dhabi, UAE

1. Introduction

There has been broad research interest in the possibility that breakfast can affect the learning and academic performance of children and adolescents.

Despite the fact that the results of these studies were diverse, breakfast intake seems to have a positive short-term effect on intellectual and cognitive performance as compared to breakfast omission in children and adolescents [2].

The definition of the term breakfast is still disputed among researchers and scientists. However, the Department of Agriculture in the United States of America has stated that the breakfast meal should contribute to at least 10% of the RDA for energy and should provide foods from at least two of the following food groups: grains, low fat dairy products, fruits, vegetables, lean meats, and finally nuts, seeds, and legumes (Lauren A. Hasz, Mark A. Lamport, 2012). Moreover, breakfast can be defined as the first meal eaten in the day before performing daily activities and it usually contributes to about 20% - 30% of total daily energy needs (Tanya Zilberter, Eugene Yuri Zilberter, 2014).

Healthy dietary practices are critical determinants of development in children and adolescents including weight status, nutritional status and cognition. One important component of a healthy diet is regular meal consumption; the consumption of breakfast has been of the greatest concern and been studied the most broadly [12].

Importantly, the American Dietary guidelines incorporate the daily consumption of a nutrient rich breakfast due to its considerable benefits [12].

Increasing breakfast consumption could be a useful public health and education enhancing intervention. However, far less research has considered the effects of breakfast on ecologically valid outcomes of academic performance compared with the relatively plentiful publications on cognitive performance. Therefore, assumptions about the benefits of breakfast for schoolchildren's learning are based on evidence demonstrating the acute effects of breakfast on schoolchildren's cognitive test performance from laboratory-based studies. The academic performance outcomes employed by studies included either school grades or standardized achievement tests. Despite the paucity of studies, there was consistent evidence that habitual breakfast consumption has a positive effect on children's academic performance. Increased frequency of habitual breakfast was consistently positively associated with academic performance [1].

The eating behaviour of individuals is affected by a large number of factors including psychological, socio-cultural and educational factors [12].

It is very critical to identify who are at higher risk of breakfast skipping and what the reasons are behind such behaviour.

Previous studies found that students with lower social economic status, lower parental educational level and divorced parents are the most likely to skip breakfast in comparison to other students [12].

Investigations found that the main reasons behind breakfast skipping among students were: not having enough time in the morning, reduced appetite, concerns about weight and body image [3].

Measurements of student performance at school have received substantial attention in earlier research; it is challenging to determine different aspects that might be of significance for student performance. There is no doubt that school performance of students is a very important factor that has a massive effect on their future. Studies found that students' school performance is dependent on a variety of factors, of which some are: quality of education, teaching methods, health and nutrition, ethnic group, age, socioeconomic status, gender, psychological factors, environmental factors and several others. These factors strongly influence student performance, but the extent of the effect may differ from individual to individual and from country to country [7].

Furthermore, studies concluded that children who are undernourished appeared to have increased absence from school and diminished attention, as well as encountering more health problems in comparison with well-nourished children, all of which would indeed affect performance at school [8].

Given the lack of studies in this area in the UAE, and due to the common practice of skipping breakfast among the young generation, more research is required in this area. Results will be valuable for health providers to develop policies and programs that focus on improving students' health and nutritional status.

Therefore, the objectives of this study were to examine the effect of breakfast intake on the academic performance of female students, to investigate some factors that lead to breakfast-skipping behaviour and to suggest possible recommendations that might encourage breakfast consumption.

2. Methods

This is a cross-sectional study where convenience sampling technique was used to select the study population. Initially a total of 150 participants, all females between the ages of 15 and 19 years, were recruited from two private schools in Abu Dhabi.

The study protocol was approved by the Research Ethics Committee at Zayed University and permission was obtained from the Abu Dhabi Education Council. Informed consent was obtained from all the students prior to their participation in the study.

Data was collected using a self-administered questionnaire to study the correlation between breakfast consumption and academic performance.

The questionnaire was developed and refined on the basis of the contents of peer review journals. It was prepared in Arabic, then translated into English and then back into Arabic and reviewed by professionals for consistency. It elicited information about breakfast intake, frequency of intake, anthropometric measurements and some demographic factors. The questionnaire was pretested and then revised to enhance its clarity and comprehension.

In order to reduce bias and ensure that the results would be as accurate and precise as possible, we chose two private the schools with the same studying hours – 7:30 in the morning to 2:30 in the afternoon – and both with the same curriculum assigned by the UAE Ministry of Education.

Out of 150 female students who agreed to participate in the study, a total of 130 were included in the study and completed the questionnaire. 9 students were excluded as they had health problems or provided incomplete answers.

The exclusion criteria included disorders or health problems that affect cognition and performance. The most common health problem that was found among students was migraines.

The academic performance of students was assessed via the grades they scored in the final exams of the first semester of the 2015-2016 academic year. As the students were studying a combination of different subjects, academic performance was assessed according to the average grade of all the subjects studied.

Data was analyzed descriptively and inferentially using the SPSS 21 software version 21 to ascertain the association between breakfast intake and academic performance. Correlation and regression were calculated and interpreted to look for any statistical significance between the variables at ≤ 0.05.

3. Results

The study sample consisted of 130 female students from the 10th, 11th and 12th grades in two schools. Their ages ranged from 15 years to 19 years, with the mean age being 16 years. Their weight ranged from 37 kg to 89 kg, with an average of 56.2 kg. Their height ranged from 145 cm to 174 cm. with an average of 160.21 cm. Body mass index (BMI) was calculated for all study subjects using appropriate formula and classification. Out of a total of 81 students who consume breakfast at least 5 times a week, 8 students were found to be underweight, 62 were within the normal weight range, 7 were overweight and 1 was obese. On the other hand, out of 49 students who regularly skip breakfast or consume it fewer than 5 times a week, 5 were found to be underweight, 32 were

Variables	N (%)
Gender	
Female	130 (100)
Age	
15	36 (27.6)
16	43 (33.1)
17	40 (30.8)
18	8 (6.2)
19	3 (2.3)
BMI	
Underweight	20 (15.4)
Normal weight	89 (68.5)
Overweight	19 (14.6)
Obese	2 (1.5)
Breakfast	
Eat (> 5 times a week)	81(62.3)
Skip (<5 times a week)	49 (37.7)
Class	
10th	46 (35.3)
11th	37 (28.5)
12th	47 (36.2)
Mean (SD)	
Age (years)	(16.2) 0.998
Weight (kg)	56.22 (9.42)
Height (cm)	160.21 (5.46)
BMI	21.79 (3.36)

TABLE 1: Descriptive characteristics of the study sample

within the normal weight range, 11 were overweight and 4 were obese. Accordingly, the average BMI for the study subjects was 21.79 (Table 1).

The correlation between breakfast intake and student score was calculated to find if there is any significant association between the two variables. The Pearson correlation coefficient was found to be 0.455. The positive value suggests that as breakfast consumption increases, the school scores increase too. The results were found to be highly significant $p < 0.001$ (Table 2).

Results of correlations		
Variables	P-value	Pearson correlation
Score	0.00	0.445
Breakfast	0.00	0.445

Table 2: The relationship between breakfast and school scores. Correlation is significant at the 0.01 level (2-tailed).

	B	Std-error	P value	95 % confidence interval for B
Class	0.416	1.358	0.760	(-2.272 - 3.103)
Age	-1.369	1.168	0.244	(-3.681 - 0.944)
BMI	-1.554	1.045	0.140	(-3.623 - 0.515)
Breakfast	6.567	1.317	0.00	(3.960 - 9.173)

Table 3: ANOVA test.

The results of further analysis based on the ANOVA test (table 3) showed that breakfast intake has a significant association with the scores as compared to other independent variables (B = 6.567). The association was found to be highly significant (p = 0.00) and it falls within the range of confidence interval (3.960 - 9.173).

As the academic performance of the study subjects was assessed via the grades they scored on the final exams, they were categorised into two goups: breakfast eaters and breakfast skippers. The grades scored by the students in the breakfast eaters group were as follows: 51.28% of the students scored A, 41.02% scored B, 7.69% scored C and 1.28% scored D. By contrast, 30.76% of the breakfast skippers group scored A, 30.76% scored B, 28,84% scored C and 9.61% scored D. None of the students in either of the groups scored F (Figure 1).

Students were asked to state the reasons that led them to skip breakfast. Many students skipped breakfast due to lack of time in the morning (37%). Other reasons for skipping breakfast reported by students were not feeling hungry (33%), not having breakfast prepared at home (15%), wanting to avoid excess weight gain (7%) and disliking the food prepared at home for breakfast (5%) (Figure 2).

4. Discussion

Recent studies revealed that breakfast consumption is highly associated with nutrition adequacy among children and adolescents [5, 9, 10]. The results of the current study provide evidence for the association between breakfast consumption and the academic performance of high school students in Abu Dhabi.

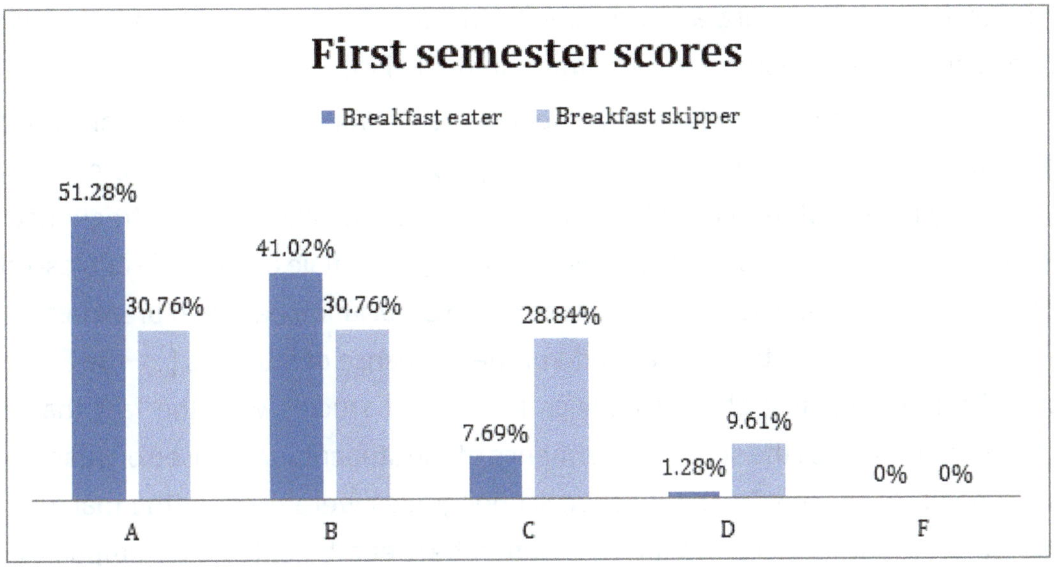

Figure 1: First semester scores.

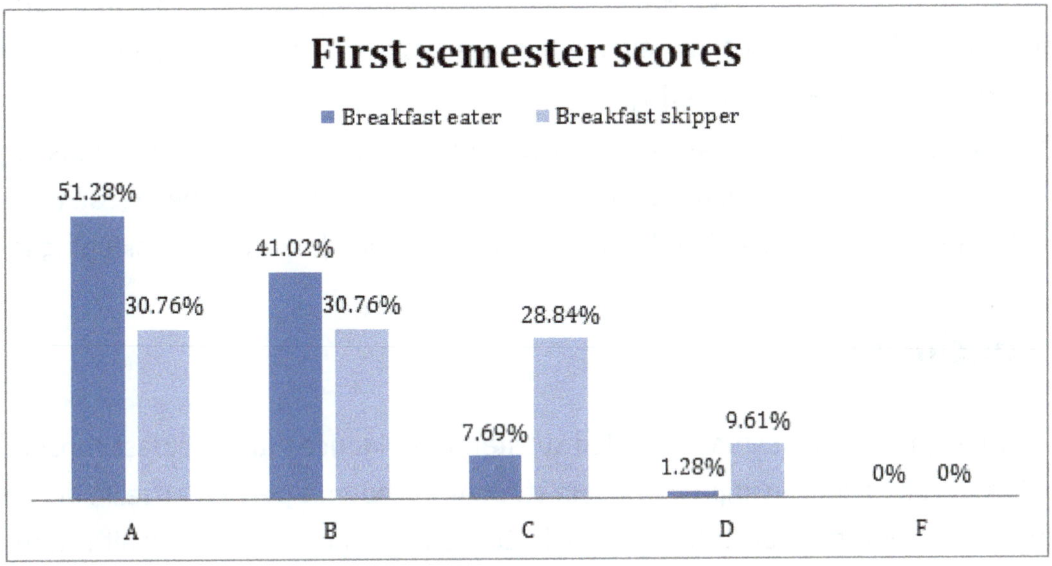

Figure 2: Reasons for breakfast skipping.

These results support the outcomes of a study that was conducted in South Korea to examine the effect of breakfast on the academic performance of both male and female adolescents from the 7th to the 12th classes. The researchers in the South Korea study were able to identify a strong link between breakfast skipping and obesity. Obesity is related to reduction in cognition and memory due to its effect on the structure of the brain. Therefore, skipping breakfast was found to be a cause for obesity, which is indeed related to lower academic performance [9].

The results of the current study also support the outcomes of the Norwegian study, which investigated the effect of a regular meal pattern on the academic performance of students. It found that the regular consumption of breakfast as well as increased intake of healthy foods are associated with increased learning outcomes and high school achievements, particularly in female students [10].

However, the association between breakfast consumption and academic performance that was revealed by the current study does not coincide with the outcomes of the study by Adolphus et al., who examined the relationship between frequency of breakfast consumption and the academic performance of male and female adolescents in the United Kingdom. The study results show no association between breakfast consumption, cognitive ability and the academic performance of students [1]. The authors justified the discrepancy of their findings from other studies with the fact that the method used to assess the school performance of the students was based on reasoning tests (Cognitive Abilities Test). However, school grades were used by the majority of other studies that investigated the association between breakfast consumption and performance including the current study.

Basch studied the negative effect of breakfast skipping on the academic performance of students. The results revealed an association between skipping breakfast and low academic performance [4].

The current study found that the most common reason for skipping breakfast was lack of time, followed by reduced appetite and not feeling hungry. These results support Affinata's results regarding the factors that might lead to breakfast skipping [3].

5. Conclusion

To conclude, the present study provided substantial evidence that breakfast consumption is associated with an improvement in students' academic performance. In drawing conclusions from this study, the Abu Dhabi Education Council and the Health Authority of Abu Dhabi should emphasize the importance of developing and implementing strategies that focus on promoting healthy eating among school-age youths and provides nutrition education guidelines for a comprehensive school health program.

These programs should target schools, parents and students with the aim of increasing knowledge of the importance of breakfast consumption and its effect on academic performance and general health. Moreover, schools and parents should look for strategies that would encourage breakfast consumption among students.

6. Acknowledgments

We would like to express our sincere gratitude to Abu Dhabi Education Council for their support to conduct this study. We are also immensely grateful to the two private schools in Abu Dhabi for their collaboration. Special thanks go to all the participants in the study, without the students' participation, this research would not have been possible.

References

[1] Adolphus K, Lawton CL and Dye L. The Relationship between Habitual Breakfast Consumption Frequency and Academic Performance in British Adolescents, Frontiers in public health 2015; 3: 68.

[2] Adolphus K, Lawton CL and Dye L. The effects of breakfast on behavior and academic performance in children and adolescents , Frontiers in human neuroscience 2013; 7: 425.

[3] Affinita A, Catalani L, Cecchetto et al. Breakfast: a multidisciplinary approach, Italian journal of pediatrics 2013; 39: 44-7288-39-44.

[4] Basch CE. Breakfast and the achievement gap among urban minority youth, The Journal of school health 2011; 81(10): 635-640.

[5] Cooper SB, Bandelow S and Nevill ME. Breakfast consumption and cognitive function in adolescent schoolchildren, Physiology and Behavior 2011; 103 (5): 431-439.

[6] Hasz LA, Lamport MA . Breakfast and Adolescent Academic Performance: An Analytical Review of Recent Research, 2015; 1 (3): 61.

[7] Mushtaq SNK. Factors Affecting Students' Academic Performance. Global Journal of Mnagment and Business Research. 2012;12 (9): 2249-4588

[8] Santanu Ghosh HS. The Role of Adequate Nutrition on Academic Performance of College Students in North Tripura 2013; 3, (3).

[9] So WY. Association between Frequency of Breakfast Consumption and Academic Performance in Healthy Korean Adolescents, Iranian journal of public health 2013; vol. 42 (1): 25-32.

[10] Stea TH and Torstveit MK. Association of lifestyle habits and academic achievement in Norwegian adolescents: a cross-sectional study, BMC public health 2014; 14: 829-2458-14-829.

[11] Zilberter T, Zilberter EY. Breakfast: To Skip or Not to Skip? 2014; 59 (2).

[12] Wijtzes AI, Jansen W, Jaddoe VW, et al. Social Inequalities in Young Children's Meal Skipping Behaviors: The Generation R Study, PloS one 2015; 10 (7): e0134487.

7

Celiac Disease or Gluten Sensitivity? A Mini Update Review

Dimitrios Papandreou

Department of Health Sciences, Zayed University, Abu Dhabi, United Arab Emirates

Corresponding Author: Dimitrios Papandreou; email: Dim-itrios.papandreou@zu.ac.ae

Abstract

Celiac disease is described when some people have with foods that contain gluten. Gluten is a type of protein. It's found in the grains wheat, barley and rye. It has antigenic properties and usually triggers an immune response. On the other hand, gluten sensitivity or intolerance is a similar condition that causes a person to react to gluten found in the above food items described. Even though the clinical symptoms are similar to both conditions, the pathology, diagnosis and treatment is different, thus it is very important to get the correct diagnosis. The purpose of this mini review is to compare the main aspects of these two conditions.

Keywords: gluten sensitivity, non celiac gluten sensitivity, celiac disease, gluten free diet

1. Introduction

The human gastrointestinal track is a very sophisticated organ that its purpose is to tolerate any antigens are coming from the external food we eat. Celiac Disease (CD) has been known for more that 2,500 years and after the half of the 20th century was linked to gluten intake. Gluten is a protein that is found in wheat, barley and rye (UC, Disease Center, 2007).

The definition of CD includes a systemic autoimmune response by the ingestion of gluten. People that are genetically susceptible to this response basically present many clinical symptoms, genetic problems with specific genes (HLA DQ2 and DQ8), increase of antigliadins (antibodies) and enteropathy [7].

In the last 20 years, the prevalence of CD has been double to almost 1% of the population [1, 6]. An explanation of this increase has been attributed to environmental factors, infections and increase consumption of wheat [15]. Predisposing factors are: age of gluten introduction, method of preparation, amount of gluten, infections in the begging of life as well as the intestinal microbiota [9]. A necessary condition to develop the disease is the presence of HLA DQ2 or DQ8 haplotype which represents about the 40% of the genetic risk [6].

Gluten is partially digested and converted to peptides rich in gliadin that when they enter the gastrointestinal cells they cause a specific immune response in the intestinal mucosa that it can lead to flattening of villi [11]. This inflammation usually spreads out to other organs such as skin and joints causing other problems not related to digestive symptoms [6].

The clinical symptoms include almost 90% in the digestive track such as diarrhea, bloating, pain, vomiting, weight loss and malnutrition [4]. Other serious symptoms include anemia, fatique, osteoporosis, headache, panic attacks, epilepsy, thyroiditis Hashimoto, type 1 Diabetes Mellitus and GI cancers [10].

The diagnosis of CD includes the presence of anti-tTG and EMA antibodies as well as the deaminated gliadin peptide antibodies (DGPs). Confirmation always requires a biopsy of the duodenum to examine and verify for any atrophy of the villi [5].

The treatment is a strict exclusion of gluten for the rest of the patient's life. A lifelong diet completely free of gluten can be very costly and challenging. Many patients' intestines don't heal completely, most often due to a failure to adhere to the gluten-free diet strictly enough.

2. Gluten Sensitivity

Non-celiac gluten sensitivity (NCGS) characterized by similar symptoms found in patients with CD. The major trigger is gluten and its pathology is still controversial, since there are a series of digestive and non-digestive symptoms (Tonnuti and Bizzaro, 2014). There are no clear number as far as concern its prevalence; however, in general population in USA, a 6% was found among 6,000 patients [14].

Except gluten other proteins such as alpha-amylase/trypsin inhibitors, and some carbohydrates (FODMAPs) may also contribute to the onset of NCGS [8]. Patients with NCGS would not activate the acquired immunity as it happens in patients with CD but innate immunity can be activated [13].

The clinical picture in NCGS patients include abdominal pain, diarrhea, fatigue, eczema, anemia, joint pain and many others and are similar to those seen in CD [3].

Differentiation with only clinical symptoms cannot be made, thus the diagnosis is made only in the absence of immune allergy response, and negative biopsy. In addition to that a gluten free diet for 3 weeks may be necessary for the resolution of the symptoms [1].

The treatment for NCGS include a gluten free diet but it does not require a strict adherence as it seen with CD patients, because there not long-term complications at this point.

3. Conclusions

Celiac Disease and gluten sensitivity share a lot of common symptoms. GD triggers the immune system while on NCGS the immune system is not activated. High levels of antibodies and positive biopsy results are common in CD and not in NCGS. Finally, both situations require a gluten free diet, CD patients need to follow that strictly for their rest of their lives while NCGS patients do not require to do that.

References

[1] C. Catassi, S. Gatti, and E. Lionetti, "World perspective and celiac disease epidemiology," *Digestive Diseases*, vol. 33, no. 2, pp. 141–146, 2015.

[2] Celiac Disease Center, A Brief History of Celiac Disease. University of Chicago, 2007, vol.7(3): pp.1-4.

[3] A. Fasano, A. Sapone, V. Zevallos, and D. Schuppan, "Nonceliac gluten sensitivity," *Gastroenterology*, vol. 148, no. 6, pp. 1195–1204, 2015.

[4] H. Garnier-Lengliné, N. Cerf-Bensussan, and F. M. Ruemmele, "Celiac disease in children," *Clinics and Research in Hepatology and Gastroenterology*, vol. 39, no. 5, pp. 544–551, 2015.

[5] K. Giersiepen, M. Lelgemann, N. Stuhldreher et al., "Accuracy of diagnostic antibody tests for coeliac disease in children: summary of an evidence report," *Journal of Pediatric Gastroenterology and Nutrition*, vol. 54, no. 2, pp. 229–241, 2012.

[6] S. Guandalini and A. Assiri, "Celiac disease: A review," *JAMA Pediatrics*, vol. 168, no. 3, pp. 272–278, 2014.

[7] S. Husby, S. Koletzko, IR. Korponay-Szabó et al., "European Society for Pediatric Gastroenterology, Hepatology, and Nutrition Guidelines for the Diagnosis of Coeliac Disease," *J Pediatr Gastroenterol Nutr*, vol. 54, no. 1, pp. 136–160, 2012.

[8] Y. Junker, S. Zeissig, S.-J. Kim et al., "Wheat amylase trypsin inhibitors drive intestinal inflammation via activation of toll-like receptor 4," *The Journal of Experimental Medicine*, vol. 209, no. 13, pp. 2395–2408, 2012.

[9] K. M. Kemppainen, K. F. Lynch, and E. Liu, "Factors that Increase Risk of Celiac Disease Autoimmunity Following a Gastrointestinal Infection in Early Life," *Clin Gastroenterol Hepatol*, vol. 15, no. 5, pp. 694–702, 2017.

[10] J. F. Ludvigsson, C. Sellgren, B. Runeson, N. Långström, and P. Lichtenstein, "Increased suicide risk in coeliac disease-a swedish nationwide cohort study," *Digestive and Liver Disease*, vol. 43, no. 8, pp. 616–622, 2011.

[11] C. Ortiz, R. Valenzuela, and A. Y. Lucero, "Celiac disease, non-celiac gluten sensitivity and wheat allergy: comparison of 3 different diseases triggered by the same food," in *Celiac disease*, vol. 88, pp. 417–423, Rev Chil Pediatr, 2017.

[12] E. Tonutti and N. Bizzaro, "Diagnosis and classification of celiac disease and gluten sensitivity," *Autoimmunity Reviews*, vol. 13, no. 4-5, pp. 472–476, 2014.

[13] A. Sapone, K. M. Lammers, G. Mazzarella et al., "Differential mucosal IL-17 expression in two gliadin-induced disorders: Gluten sensitivity and the autoimmune enteropathy celiac disease," *International Archives of Allergy and Immunology*, vol. 152, no. 1, pp. 75–80, 2010.

[14] A. Sapone, J. C. Bai, C. Ciacci et al., "Spectrum of gluten-related disorders: consensus on new nomenclature and classification," *BMC Medicine*, vol. 10, article 13, 2012.

[15] L. E. White, V. M. Merrick, E. Bannerman et al., "The rising incidence of celiac disease in Scotland," *Pediatrics*, vol. 132, no. 4, pp. e924–e931, 2013.

8

Review of Health Literacy and Nutrition-Related Research in the Middle East

Ludmilla F. Wikkeling-Scott[1] and R.V. Rikard[2]

[1]Assistant Professor, Zayed University, College of Natural and Health Sciences, Department of Health Sciences
[2]Senior Postdoctoral Research Associate, Michigan State University, Department of Media and Information

Corresponding Author: Ludmilla F. Wikkeling-Scott; email: Ludmilla.scott@zu.ac.ae

Abstract

Aim: In the Middle East where nutrition-related diseases continue to be on the rise, health literacy related research may provide meaningful insight to patient-provider communication, nutrition and general health behavior, to improve health outcomes. Yet, little is known about health literacy in the region. We provide insight into the current research on health literacy and nutrition-related outcomes in the region. **Methods:** English-language articles were identified using relevant keywords to search PubMed, Medline, Web of Science, and ProQuest Middle East & African. Inclusion criteria were quantitative and qualitative studies of any design focused on health literacy and nutrition-related health outcomes in the Middle East. We identified 22 unduplicated articles that met inclusion criteria. **Results:** To date, only three studies employ a validated health literacy measure to examine the relationship between health literacy and nutrition-related disease outcomes (e.g., diabetes, overweight, and obesity). However, the research findings from the three studies cannot be generalized to larger populations within each country. Participants were patients who regularly visited health care facilities. The limited samples may bias conclusions regarding health literacy and the influence on nutrition-related disease outcomes. **Conclusions:** Research is needed to understand health literacy and health literacy needs in Middle East countries, which are known for their racial and ethnic, and socio-economic diversity. Researchers can take advantage of the multitude of health literacy tools which have been validated and are readily available for use in diverse populations. Established health literacy measures provide greater benefit than developing brand new assessments when important information is urgently needed to address nutrition-related health outcomes.

Keywords: Health literacy, Nutrition-related health outcomes, Middle East, commentary

1. Introduction

In two decades, the Middle East has seen a drastic change in nutrition related health issues due to demographic and economic growth [2]. Most countries in this region can attribute an overflow of high-energy dietary products and affluence to such issues as diabetes, overweight, obesity, and cardiovascular disease; while a few countries experience nutrition insecurity [19]. Although low rates of malnutrition occur in Morocco and the United Arab Emirates; high levels of malnutrition are a major contributor to stunted childhood development in other countries such as Yemen [25].

Health literacy is a key predictor of health outcomes. Health literacy is the degree to which individuals have the capacity to obtain, process, and understand basic health information and services needed to make appropriate health decisions [15]. Health literacy is a different concept than literacy, which is the ability to use printed and written information to function in society and to achieve one's goals [9]. Variations of the definition of health literacy exist; but researchers agree that health literacy is important and influences health promotion, health care utilization, and health outcomes [24].

A growing body of health literacy research emerged from North America, Europe, Asia, and Australia [8, 24]. A number of countries recognize health literacy as a priority [1]. Outside of the United States (U.S.) an increasing international body of health literacy research developed over the past decade [18]. However, little research exists to understand the health literacy needs of people in the Middle East. Nutrition-related illness and the dependence on health care intervention are cause for health literacy interventions. However, there is a wide gap in studies examining health literacy and nutrition-related health outcomes for the Middle East [23]. Our aim is to shed some light on health literacy and nutrition-related health outcome research in the Middle East. Specifically, we examine the types and location (i.e., country) of studies examining health literacy in the context of nutrition-related health outcomes.

2. Attributes of Health Literacy

Health literacy has two main attributes: functional and complex skills. The first, functional health literacy skills, includes the ability to obtain health information, demonstrate basic reading skills, and understand health information. The second component, complex skills, is needed to fully utilize information obtained, and interact with health care providers and within health care systems. This implies a shared responsibility between individuals and health care providers to achieve levels of adequate health literacy and ultimately achieve successful outcomes for a health care need [4, 9]. Thus, health literacy is not any one person's problem, it is a collective effort to achieve health outcomes and a critical component of overall health care. Health literacy skills need to be included in nutrition-related interventions to change health outcomes, but in the Middle East there is little evidence of this.

3. Health Literacy Gap

The National Academy of Medicine (formerly the Institute of Medicine) reported that up to 50% of adults lack the literacy skills needed to function adequately in a health care environment [27]. Some research suggests an association between health literacy and increased hospitalization, but no universal consensus has yet been established [7, 14]. Persons with low levels of health literacy may often feel embarrassed due to inadequate language skills, and may need motivation to access health care resources and gain confidence to navigate the increasingly complex health care systems [16].

Language barriers and lack of culturally competent services within the modern and often complex health care systems may create obstacles for achieving adequate health literacy [22]. Persons with low levels of health literacy may often feel embarrassed due to inadequate language skills and may need support to access health care resources and gain confidence to navigate the systems [16]. Different countries may define health literacy in other terms such as health awareness, health communication, health promotion, health beliefs, and communication for healthy living, wherefore the term health literacy may seem unfamiliar [4]. Some research shows that health care providers may not be equipped to understand and deal with cultural differences, which may affect patient-provider communication in understanding seriousness of disease, management of disease, health status and treatment options [23]. Studies show evidence of a significant relationship between health literacy, health outcomes, health care utilization and health care spending [5, 21].

4. Methods

Two researchers independently conducted a systematic search and review in four databases, namely: ProQuest Middle East & Africa database, Medline, PubMed, Web of Science, and Google Scholar during the Spring and Summer of 2017. Results were then compared and combined to obtain information to interpret research on health outcomes associated with nutrition behavior and related health literacy research activities, in the Middle East. The research teams first searched for relevant studies readily identifiable for health literacy by country, and then applied supplementary search strategies to relevant electronic databases.

4.1. Inclusion Criteria

We considered studies of any design which examined relationships between health literacy (assessed by validated existing and or new instruments) or health-related knowledge or behaviors and nutrition-related health outcomes in Middle East population whose first language was the dominant language of their resident country. Studies were included if: 1) their description and or use of a definition for health literacy or a newly established definition relevant to the local country/region was evident in their investigation of nutrition-related health outcomes, 2) a health literacy focus was evident, and 3) the study offered relevant content and a framework for developing hypotheses relayed to health literacy in the context of nutrition-related health outcomes. Eligible studies were then tallied and separated by country, study design, and health literacy assessment instrument.

4.2. Search Strategy

The search for readily identifiable health literacy research in the Middle East was conducted using the key terms "health" AND "literacy" AND "name of each country listed in Table 1. Although the search term, health literacy, was common to the search strategy, adjustments were made to take advantage of the different indexing terms available within individual databases. Additional searches included the terms "health" AND "awareness," "communication," "promotion," "beliefs", and "communication for healthy living" to take into consideration the possible interchange of terminology among researchers in the Middle East.

5. Results

The results describe the region of the Middle East, countries included and the main language(s) spoken (Table 1). A review of data by country on health literacy research in the context of nutrition-related health outcomes in the region considered as the Middle East (Table 2). Differences exist in the list of member-countries which are considered a part of the Middle East. Results showed that those countries listed in Table 1 were appropriately labeled as member countries. Twenty countries were identified as member countries of the Middle East. The four-member countries of Algeria, Libya,

Country	Primary Language(s)
Algeria	Arabic
Bahrain	Arabic
Egypt	Arabic/Egyptian
Iran	Persian
Iraq	Arabic/Kurdish
Israel	Arabic/Hebrew
Jordan	Arabic
Kuwait	Arabic
Lebanon	Arabic
Libya	Arabic
Morocco	Arabic
Oman	Arabic
Qatar	Arabic
Saudi Arabia	Arabic
Syria	Arabic
The Palestinian Territories	Arabic
Tunisia	Arabic
Turkey	Turkish
United Arab Emirates	Arabic
Yemen	Arabic

TABLE 1: Middle Eastern Countries and Primary Language.

Morocco and Tunisia are located in Northeast Africa and are considered part of the Middle East due to cultural ties and Arabic as the national language. Another country on the African continent, Egypt, also Arabic-speaking, has historically played a political role in the Middle East and is considered a member of the region.

Among member countries, two are non-Arabic-speaking, namely Iran, where the national language is Persian and Turkey, where the national language is Turkish. While three countries are recognized for as bilingual national language users, namely: Egypt (Arabic and Egyptian), Iraq (Arabic and Kurdish), and Israel (Arabic and Hebrew). Health literacy research has only been conducted in 10 Middle Eastern countries. However, we describe only studies related to health literacy and nutrition-related health outcomes. Among the countries that have conducted health literacy research, only three of the

Country	Author(s) & Year	Purpose	Study Design	Health Literacy Assessment	Sample	Results
Iran	[10]	To identify the effect of various factors on health literacy in patients with diabetes.	Cross-Sectional	TOFHLA - Persian	N = 407	Health literacy not associated with HbA1c.
					38.3% males	
					61.7% females	
Iran	[20]	To document the relationships between functional, communicative, and critical health literacy, self-efficacy, outcome expectations, and diabetes self-care of patients with type 2 diabetes mellitus (T2DM) in Iran.	Cross-Sectional	The multi-dimensional scale of Functional Communicative and Critical Health Literacy (FCCHL)	N = 187	Positive and significant association between communicative and critical health literacy, self-efficacy, and diabetes self-care management. Functional health literacy not significant with self-care management.
					32.1% males	
					67.9% females	
Saudi Arabia	Al-Ruthia, Y. S., Balkhi, B., AlGhadeer, S., Mansy, W., AlSanawi, H., AlGasem, R., & Sales, I. (2017).	Relationship between health literacy and body mass index among Arab women with polycystic ovary syndrome.	Cross-Sectional	Single Item Literacy Screener (SILS)	N=127	Higher BMI significant lower likelihood of good health literacy.
					100% females	

TABLE 2: Research on Health Literacy and Nutrition-Related Health Outcomes in the Middle East.

studies focused on nutrition-related health outcomes (Table 2), two in Iran and 1 in Saudi Arabia.

The studies focused on 1) the association between health literacy and body mass index (BMI) among polycystic ovarian syndrome patients, 2) the effect of varying levels of health literacy on diabetes-related outcomes, and 3) the relationship between health literacy and diabetes self-management. One of the studies was gender specific, while the other two studies had less than 40% male participation. Two studies used a health literacy measure or tool from the health literacy toolshed [3], which is a database for research on validated health literacy measures published in peer-reviewed journals.

The Arabic version of the single item literacy screener (SILS) [11] identified patients in Saudi-Arabia with low health literacy. This tool was first validated and published in 2006, in the United States, among 97% White and 3% other racial and ethnic groups of diabetes patients, in a region-wide sample, representative of the state population. The SILS is designed to identify persons with limited reading ability and in need of assistance navigating written health-related information. The Saudi-Arabian study sample consisted of 127 women with an average age of 27.40 years, and indicated that 16.54% of participants had limited health literacy. The study suggests patients with limited health literacy are more likely to have higher BMI. The study concluded that future studies are necessary to examine health-literacy enhancing interventions that can influence disease outcome.

The Iranian version of the multidimensional of Functional Communicative and Critical Health Literacy (FCCHL) [6, 20] scale was used to describe the relationship between health literacy, self-efficacy, outcome expectations, and diabetes self-care of patients with type 2 diabetes mellitus (T2DM) in Iran. This tool was first validated and published in 2008, in Japan, among diabetes patients, visiting a single hospital, and familiar with their health care provider. The tool is intended to measure three aspects of health literacy, functional, communicative and critical. The Iranian study sample consisted of 187 patients, 80.5% married, 67.9% female, and 57.2% had a primary education. Patients who received diabetes education and were married had better diabetes self-care behavior. Communicative and critical health literacy levels were found to be significantly higher in married participants. Low health literacy was related to increased age and low educational levels. The authors conclude that communicative and critical health literacy are an attribute of self-efficacy and self-care activities. The authors further suggests the use of health literacy for identifying barriers to self-efficacy in management of diabetes, which may be related to nutrition-behavior [13].

The Iranian version of the Test of Functional Health Literacy in Adults (TOFHLA) identified the effects of various factors on health literacy in diabetes patients in a single university based diabetes clinic [10, 17]. The tool was first validated and published in 1995 in the United States, among English- and Spanish-speaking patients in two outpatient settings in public hospitals. The Iranian study sample consisted of 470 patients, 61.7% female, and 85.9% married with significant differences lower educational levels among females as compared to males. Results suggested a positive relationship between level of education, employment and health literacy. The results showed 70% of participants had inadequate health literacy levels and a correlation between reading comprehension, and numeracy skills. This study results showed an inverse relationship between level of health literacy and age: the older the patient, the lower the level of health literacy. There was no significant relationship between health literacy and levels of HbA1c. The study suggests the design of effective interventions to improve diabetes-related outcomes.

6. Discussion

Our aim is to describe research activities examining health literacy and nutrition-related disease outcomes. Health literacy, although popular in Western countries, Asia, and Australia has yet to find a solid base in the Middle East. Few studies exist and although multiple tools are available, few researchers take advantage of the existing evidence to understand health literacy and health literacy needs in the Middle East. Only three studies were identified relating health literacy to nutrition-related disease outcome measures. Dramatic increases in chronic disease rates, attributed to nutrition behavior, warrant more intense investigation into the role of health literacy in disease outcomes. Health literacy is a well-established and critical component of disease prevention and imperative for successful health promotion.

The three studies identified, were very specific in their focus, in that they targeted persons familiar with chronic disease only. The settings in each of the studies might have decreased the usability of the results due to the sample size and location, and limited knowledge of general health literacy levels in the population.

Health literacy in chronic disease patients tends to be higher than in other communities, due to the fact that these persons regularly engage with health care providers and are forced to deal with more health information to manage disease [26].

The current studies are not generalizable due to their specificity in sample and location, and use of study tools. The health literacy toolshed is a starting point for those communities where health literacy has not yet been measured to assess community needs. However, this toolshed may also be a good starting point for research in specific populations, when no other research for that population exists to validate the tools locally and describe health literacy needs. Health literacy is a process, wherefore it is not only useful to understand the picture in sub-populations with very specific characteristics, but for those who may or may not ever be included in such populations. An example is the population of young adolescents and young adults, who are becoming more vulnerable to poor nutrition-related health outcomes. Increased access to the internet, with massive nutrition information, and changing cultural habits may influence health outcomes in younger populations. Access to care, increased government support to fund health care services and availability of health care services may enable persons to avoid self-management and seek health care provider help instead. Many Middle East countries are known to have a high number of expatriate health care providers compared to the number of local workforce. Cultural and language issues in health care and health literacy needs for the health care system, must be considered.

Environmental factors, such as year-round dry heat, time spent indoors provides a great opportunity for consumption of a multitude of fast food choices and pre-cooked foods, and a lack of physical activity. Inherent in a majority of the culture in the region, is the large consumption of tobacco product, which is considered one of the top non-dietary risk factors affecting health outcomes in the Middle East [12]. Undernutrition is a risk for vulnerable populations in the region, while the shift from traditional to a more diverse diet rich in carbohydrates, proteins, saturated and trans fats, sugar and salt also increases poor health outcomes for the region [19].

7. Conclusion

Several factors contribute to the increasing rates of nutrition-related chronic disease and strategies to address the gap in knowledge about health literacy as a key indicator of health outcomes. To begin addressing the burden of chronic disease on the region, we must first understand the characteristics of communities and sub-communities affected, and their specific needs in order to effectively design health literacy interventions for countries in the region. More research is needed to begin interpreting health literacy needs regionally and by country.

As a starting point, countries in the region should actively build awareness for individuals, health care providers, and other stakeholders that will precede health promotions activities (Adams et al., 2009). A conceptual model for health literacy in the context of nutrition-related health promotions should be aimed at improving knowledge and understanding of health determinants, and improving nutrition behavior. The relatively young population representing diverse countries in the Middle East can be targeted in school systems, to create awareness and the need for physical activity coupled with nutrition education. By including the educational system, a partnership to develop health literacy initiatives from a non-clinical perspective can be developed.

One limitation may be the lack of community health and practices linked only to clinical settings, which may limit nutrition-related health promotions activities to merely those conducted in collaboration with or in clinical settings. A community-based approach linking individuals, health care providers, policymakers, and stakeholders, will be the challenge to prescribe health literacy as a key indicator of nutrition-related and other disease outcomes.

References

[1] R. H. Carmona, "Health literacy: a national priority," *Journal of General Internal Medicine*, vol. 21, no. 8, p. 803, 2006.

[2] O. Galal, "Nutrition-related health patterns in the Middle East," *Asia Pacific Journal of Clinical Nutrition*, vol. 12, no. 3, pp. 337–343, 2003.

[3] S. Harnett, "Health Literacy Tool Shed: A Source for Validated Health Literacy Instruments," *Journal of Consumer Health on the Internet*, vol. 21, no. 1, pp. 78–86, 2017.

[4] J. Hatamleh and M. Huff, "Health literacy of Iraqi immigrant adults: pilot study," *International Journal of Healthcare*, vol. 2, no. 1, 2015.

[5] D. H. Howard, J. Gazmararian, and R. M. Parker, "The impact of low health literacy on the medical costs of Medicare managed care enrollees," *American Journal of Medicine*, vol. 118, no. 4, pp. 371–377, 2005.

[6] H. Ishikawa, T. Takeuchi, and E. Yano, "Measuring functional, communicative, and critical health literacy among diabetic patients," *Diabetes Care*, vol. 31, no. 5, pp. 874–879, 2008.

[7] S. Kim, F. Love, D. A. Quistberg, and J. A. Shea, "Association of health literacy with self-management behavior in patients with diabetes," *Diabetes Care*, vol. 27, no. 12, pp. 2980–2982, 2004.

[8] B. K. Kondilis, I. J. Kiriaze, A. P. Athanasoulia, and M. E. Falagas, "Mapping health literacy research in the European Union: A bibliometric analysis," *PLoS ONE*, vol. 3, no. 6, Article ID e2519, 2008.

[9] M. Kutner, E. Greenburg, Y. Jin, and C. Paulsen, *The health literacy of america's adults: Results from the 2003 national assessment of adult literacy*, U.S. Department of Education, Washington, 2006.

[10] Z. Mohammadi, A. T. Banihashemi, H. Asgharifard, M. Bahramian, H. R. Baradaran, and M. E. Khamseh, "Health literacy and its influencing factors in Iranian diabetic patients," *Medical Journal of The Islamic Republic of Iran*, vol. 29, no. 1, article no. 230, 2015.

[11] N. S. Morris, C. D. MacLean, L. D. Chew, and B. Littenberg, "The Single Item Literacy Screener: Evaluation of a brief instrument to identify limited reading ability," *BMC Family Practice*, vol. 7, article no. 21, 2006.

[12] A. O. Musaiger, "Overweight and obesity in the Eastern Mediterranean Region: Can we control it?" *Eastern Mediterranean Health Journal*, vol. 10, no. 6, pp. 789–793, 2004.

[13] S. W. Ng, S. Zaghloul, H. I. Ali, G. Harrison, and B. M. Popkin, "The prevalence and trends of overweight, obesity and nutrition-related non-communicable diseases in the Arabian Gulf States," *Obesity Reviews*, vol. 12, no. 1, pp. 1–13, 2011.

[14] C. Y. Osborn, B. D. Weiss, T. C. Davis et al., "Measuring adult literacy in health care: performance of the newest vital sign," *American Journal of Health Behavior*, vol. 31, suppl. 1, pp. S36–S46, 2007.

[15] R. Parker, "Health literacy: A challenge for American patients and their health care providers," *Health Promotion International*, vol. 15, no. 4, pp. 277–283, 2000.

[16] R. Parker and S. C. Ratzan, "Health literacy: A second decade of distinction for Americans," *Journal of Health Communication*, vol. 15, no. 2, pp. 20–33, 2010.

[17] R. M. Parker, D. W. Baker, M. V. Williams, and J. R. Nurss, "The test of functional health literacy in adults: a new instrument for measuring patients' literacy skills," *Journal of General Internal Medicine*, vol. 10, no. 10, pp. 537–541, 1995.

[18] A. Pleasant, *Health literacy around the world: Part 1. Health literacy efforts outside of the united states*, National Academies Press, Washington, D.C., 2013.

[19] B. M. Popkin and P. Gordon-Larsen, "The nutrition transition: Worldwide obesity dynamics and their determinants," *International Journal of Obesity*, vol. 28, pp. S2–S9, 2004.

[20] M. Reisi, F. Mostafavi, H. Javadzade, B. Mahaki, E. Tavassoli, and G. Sharifirad, "Impact of health literacy, self-efficacy, and outcome expectations on adherence to self-care behaviors in iranians with type 2 diabetes," *Oman Medical Journal*, vol. 31, no. 1, pp. 52–59, 2016.

[21] D. Schillinger, K. Grumbach, J. Piette et al., "Association of health literacy with diabetes outcomes," *Journal of the American Medical Association*, vol. 288, no. 4, pp. 475–482, 2002.

[22] P. M. Schyve, "Language differences as a barrier to quality and safety in health care: The joint commission perspective," *Journal of General Internal Medicine*, vol. 22, no. 2, pp. 360–361, 2007.

[23] S. J. Shaw, C. Huebner, J. Armin, K. Orzech, and J. Vivian, "The role of culture in health literacy and chronic disease screening and management," *Journal of Immigrant and Minority Health*, vol. 11, no. 6, pp. 460–467, 2009.

[24] K. Sørensen, S. Van Den Broucke, J. Fullam et al., "Health literacy and public health: A systematic review and integration of definitions and models," *BMC Public Health*, vol. 12, no. 1, article no. 80, 2012.

[25] T. S. Sunil, "Effects of socio-economic and behavioural factors on childhood malnutrition in Yemen," *Maternal & Child Nutrition*, vol. 5, no. 3, pp. 251–259, 2009.

[26] E. H. Wagner, R. E. Glasgow, C. Davis et al., "Quality improvement in chronic illness care: a collaborative approach," *Community Journal of Quality Improvement*, vol. 27, pp. 63–79, 2001.

[27] B. D. Weiss, M. Z. Mays, W. Martz et al., "Quick assessment of literacy in primary care: the newest vital sign," *Annals of Family Medicine*, vol. 3, no. 6, pp. 514–522, 2005.

9

A Study on Foodborne Bacterial Cross-contamination During Fresh Chicken Preparation

Shamma Ebrahim AlZaabi[1] and Munawwar Ali Khan[2]

[1]Health and Safety Department, UAE Armed Forces, GHQ, Abu Dhabi, United Arab Emirates
[2]Department of Life and Environmental Sciences, College of Natural and Health Sciences, Zayed University, P.O. Box: 19282, Dubai, United Arab Emirates

Corresponding Author: Munawwar Ali Khan; email: Munawwar.Khan@zu.ac.ae

Abstract

Background: Cross-contamination of foodborne pathogens from undercooked poultry meat to ready-to-eat food has been shown to be responsible for a number of foodborne disease outbreaks. Various studies have indicated that bacterial cross-contamination occurs during food preparation where bacteria present on food contact other surfaces and cause illness. **Objectives:** This study evaluated the ability of bacteria to survive and cross-contaminate other foods during the preparation of fresh chicken. *Salmonella spp.* cross-contamination from chicken to cucumber and utensils under various food handling scenarios was determined. **Methods:** Two scenarios were tested: in scenario 1, cutting board and knife used for cutting chicken without washing step were sampled. In scenario 2, cutting board and knife was washed with tap water separately after cutting chicken, and subsequently used for cutting cucumber. In scenario 1, chicken, cutting board, knife, and hands were sampled, and in scenario 2, cucumber was tested. Fluorescent *in situ* hybridization (FISH) method, using published Salmonella specific gene probes was used for *Salmonella* detection in samples taken from cross-contamination scenarios. A culture-based detection by Hektoen enteric agar was used for the confirmation of *Salmonella* species. **Results:** All the samples analyzed were found to be positive for *Salmonella spp.* with different contamination levels. These results were further confirmed by culture based method. In scenario 1, *Salmonella spp.* was detected by Sal-1 and Salm-63 oligonucleotide probes in all four samples (chicken, cutting board, knife and hands). A high contamination level was observed in chicken samples in comparison to samples collected from cutting board, knife and hands. In scenario 2, *Salmonella spp.* was detected by Sal-1 and Salm-63 oligonucleotide probes in the cucumber with very low contamination level. *Salmonella Enterica* was also detected by Sal-3 and Sapath-3 in both scenarios but the contamination level was not high as compared to *Salmonella spp.* **Conclusion:** In conclusion, *Salmonella spp.* cross-contamination during fresh chicken preparation to read-to-eat-food (cucumber) was confirmed by this study. The experimental data obtained in this study clearly suggest that it is extremely difficult to prevent the spread of *Salmonella spp.* during the preparation of raw poultry-based meals. Therefore, extreme precautions such as proper cleaning and sanitization of utensils, equipment and surfaces should be carefully followed during the preparation of fresh poultry meat-based food items.

Keywords: Cross-contamination; foodborne pathogens; *Salmonella*; chicken

1. Introduction

The importance of food for human health has been widely recognized; eating safe food and optimal quantities of nutritious is a basic human right and a major precondition for a happy and productive life [17]. Therefore, the prevention of diseases and improvement of human health is of paramount significance, not only for governments but also for consumers themselves. Additionally, the production of safe food is based on the implementation of general preventive measures such as Good Hygiene Practices (GHP) and such application of measure represents the pre-requisite conditions required in preparing safe food [18, 19]. Cross contamination is a general term which refers to the transfer, direct or indirect, of bacteria or viruses from a contaminated product or surfaces to non-contaminated products" [2]. Cross contamination plays a significant role in transferring harmful pathogens such as *Campylobacter* and *Salmonella* to fresh produce [5, 16, 22].

Several studies have been conducted in households' kitchen settings to determine the effect of microbial cross-contamination via chopping board, cutlery, and hands on the microbiological quality of a realistically prepared meal ready to eat food [4, 6, 12, 20]. These and several other closely related studies indicated that microbial contamination of kitchen surfaces during food preparation due to foodborne bacteria present in foodstuff is one of the main causes of foodborne outbreaks. Many investigators revealed that bacteria cells adhered to those surfaces of domestic kitchens are not easily removed by normal cleaning procedures [3, 5, 22] and various pathogenic bacteria like *Campylobacter and Salmonella* survive in kitchen utensils, hands and possibly cross contaminate other food Several studies indicate that various pathogenic bacteria like *Campylobacter and Salmonella* survive in kitchen utensils, hands and possibly cross contaminate other food [7, 13, 21]. Therefore, it is very important to understand the adhesion of pathogenic bacteria to kitchen utensils that are used in the preparation of meal. Microbial contamination, can be easily passed from kitchen items to the food when contacting food, this normally happens when equipments are not efficiently cleaned and sanitized between each use [5, 22]. Microbial contamination from food to food occurs mainly when raw foods, especially poultry meat comes into contact with cooked or ready to eat foods through chopping board and contaminated utensils [11, 13]. A number of survey studies have reported on the unsafe practices common among consumers in the kitchen [5, 16]. Because of the inefficient use of cutting surfaces, as well as the applied cleaning methods may lead to the cross contamination of ready to eat food with the *Salmonella* spp.

As indicated in the several studies published over the past several years that food-borne illness remains a significant worldwide problem, and cross-contamination is believed to play a key role in the transmission of foodborne pathogens, especially *Salmonella* spp., which is one of the major causative organisms for the food-borne diarrheal disease locally and globally [2, 20]. The transfer of *Salmonella* is possible from naturally contaminated chicken to different cutting surfaces and then to cucumber handled on the common food cutting surfaces, as these kinds of food practices are very common in the household conditions. The present study was designed to closely mimic the cross-contamination scenarios of *Salmonella* from naturally contaminated fresh chicken to ready to eat food (cucumber) via cutting board, knife, and gloved hands. Two cross contamination scenarios were simulated, and Fluorescent *in situ* hybridization (FISH) and culture based methods were used to evaluate *Salmonella* cross contamination in this study. *Salmonella* spp. is the foodborne bacteria, which was chosen as a model bacterium in this study, as it belongs to the most foodborne bacteria causing infections worldwide. The main objective of the study was to evaluate the ability of *Salmonella* spp. to survive and cross-contaminate ready to eat food (cucumber) during the preparation of fresh chicken.

2. Materials and Methods

2.1. Sample Collection

The fresh chicken carcass was purchased from the slaughterhouse on the same day of the experiment to increase the probability of obtaining a true Salmonella positive sample and to decrease the chance of contamination and subsequent false positive results. The chicken carcass obtained from the slaughterhouse was immediately placed in a plastic bag and transported to the microbiology laboratory in an ice filled container. The sample was processed within one hour of being collected. Fresh and damage-free cucumber was also brought from the market. Clean and sterilized cutting board and knife were placed in the lab as well.

2.2. Cross-Contamination Scenarios

To evaluate the cross-contamination of *Salmonella*, two different cross-contamination scenarios were simulated. The experiment started with sterilizing the location of the experiment by using 70% of ethanol. The cutting board and knife were scrubbed and rinsed thoroughly using commercial detergent and tap water, and then dried thoroughly with paper towels. Sterile Gloves were used throughout the experiment and 70% ethanol was used for further sterilization of hands. The following scenarios were tested.

2.3. Scenario 1 (Cross-Contamination of Cutting Board, Knife Blade and Hands)

The chicken sample was placed on the detergent washed cutting board. The chicken was first sampled directly before preparation by using sterile cotton swabs. This sampling was done based on preliminary experiments which have shown that all parts of the chicken have approximately equal number of bacterial load [12]. Thus, the sampling of the chicken was taken from different parts of the chicken, assuming that each part carried the same number of bacteria. The household kitchen scenario was simulated for the preparation of chicken by cutting chicken into small pieces with a detergent sterilized knife. The chicken pieces were turned once to simulate the amount of handling. Afterwards, the cutting board, the blade of the knife and both hands were sampled (Fig. 1).

2.4. Scenario 2 (Cross-Contamination of Cucumber)

A similar experiment as the one described above was conducted, with the exception that after simulating the preparation of chicken in scenario 1, the gloves were changed and both hands were washed thoroughly with soap and tap water, and then dried with paper towels. The cutting board and knife were rinsed just with tap water without using commercial detergent. Therefore, cutting board and knife remained unsterilized. Fresh cucumber was placed on the cutting board after rinsing it by tap water, and cut into pieces using the knife. This was to simulate the slicing of salad ingredients (cucumber) without sterilizing the cutting board and knife. The cucumber slices were then sampled by using sterile cotton swabs (Fig. 1). In total ten samples obtained from the 2 cross contamination scenarios were used for detection of *Salmonella*.

2.5. Detection of Salmonella Species

Molecular-based method such as fluorescent *in situ* hybridization (FISH) is a sensitive and robust assay applied for whole-cell detection via hybridization with nucleic acids within the target cell and without altering the morphological integrity of the cells [23].

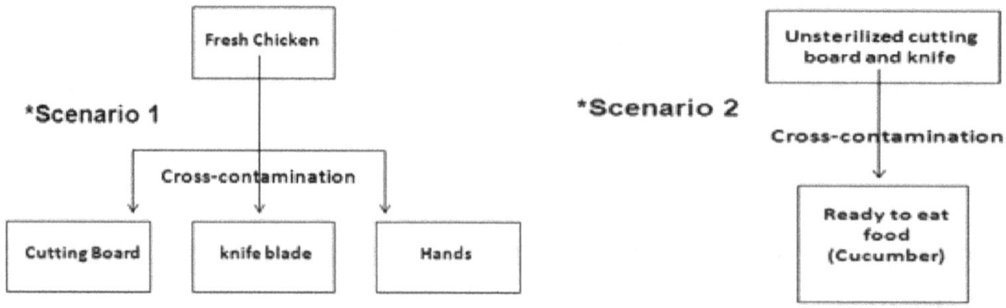

Figure 1: Cross-contamination scenarios determined in this study.

FISH is based on the hybridization of a genomic sequence characteristic of food-borne bacteria which specifically immobilized and label whole bacterial cells by fluorescently labeled rRNA oligonucleotide probes [1]. FISH assay was performed on obtained samples by following these common steps: fixation, sample preparation, hybridization of the probe and the target sequence, washing off the excess unbound probe and finally detecting and visualizing the labeled cells by the application fluorescent microscopy as described previously [14, 15]. Four oligonucleotide probes were used: two *Salmonella* spp. probe, Sal1 [10], Salm-63 [9]; a *Salmonella enterica* oligonucleotide probe, Sal-3 [15]; the *Salmonella enteric* subsp. probe (Sapath3) [10]. For further detection and confirmation of the presence of *Salmonella*, classical culture based method was preformed to support the results obtained from the rapid detection by FISH assay. Selective and differential agar (Hektoen Enteric Agar) was used to isolate and differentiate *Salmonella*. The swab samples from Chicken, cutting board, knife, hands and cucumber were streaked onto the surface of the plates. The plates were incubated for 24-48 hours and then viewed to check for growth of dark greenish colonies of *Salmonella*.

3. Results and Discussion

The hybridization conditions for the oligonucleotide probes used in this study (Sal1, Sal3, Salm-63 and Sapath3) were optimized to obtain a positive fluorescence signal for the detection of previously isolated *Salmonella* strains from the chicken samples [8]. These probes gave negative results with the non-target organisms. In most cases, hybridization with Sal1, Sal3, and Sapath3 probes showed best possible fluorescence signal, when 25% formamide was used in the hybridization solution. However, 35% formamide concentration was found to be the best for the Salm-63 probe. The results of FISH based analysis of the samples obtained from two cross contamination scenarios are summarized in table 1.

Samples	Oligonucleotide probes used for the detection of Salmonella			
	Sal1 (*Salmonella* spp)	**Sal3** *(Salmonella enterica)*	**Salm-63** (*Salmonella* spp)	**Sapath3** (*Salmonella enteric* subsp)
	25% of formamide	25% of formamide	35% of formamide	25% of formamide
CK	+++	+/-	+++	+++
B	++	++	++	++
K	+	+	+	+
H	+++	++	++	+++
Cucm	+/-	++	+/-	+++

TABLE 1: Detection of *Salmonella* in samples of food handling scenarios by FISH technique. *Abbreviation used: **CK:** Chicken, **B:** Cutting Board, **K:** Knife, **H:** Hands, **Cucm:** Cucumber, **(+++):** Signal with high contamination, **(++):** Signal with moderate contamination, **(+):** Signal with low contamination, **(+/-):** Contamination with weak signal.

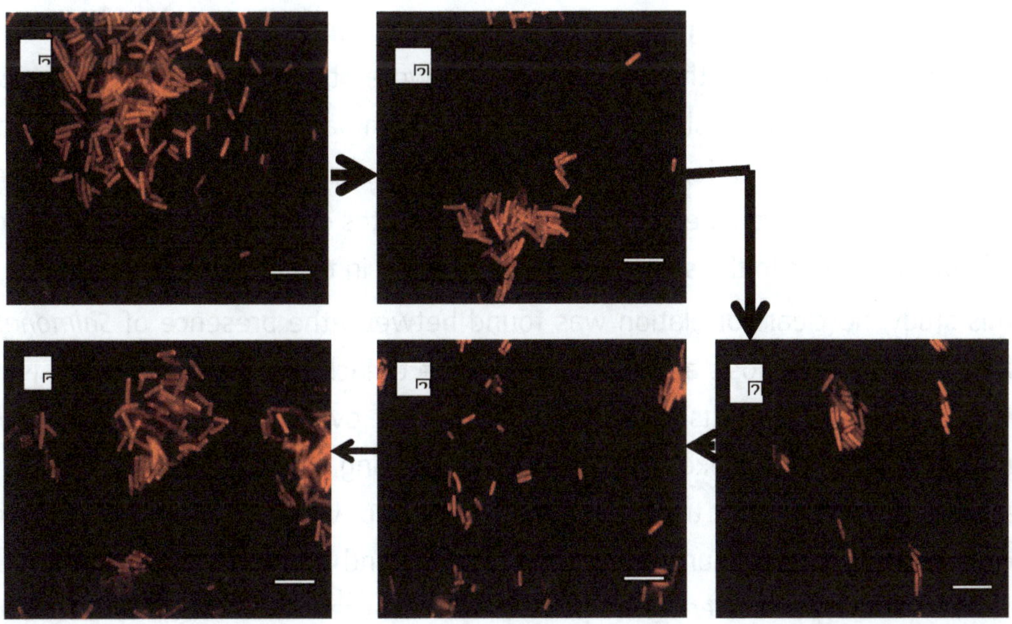

Figure 2: In situ hybridization of samples (chicken, cutting board, Knife, hands and cucumber): *Salmonella* species hybridized by TRITC-labeled Sal-1 probe. **A)** Chicken sample; **B)** Cutting board; **C)** Knife; **D)** Hands; **E)** Cutting board. Bar =10 μm and applies to all photomicrographs. Original magnification: 1000X.

All oligonucleotide probes included in this study detected *Salmonella* in all samples directly obtained from the five items. The probes Sal3 and Sapath3 were specifically hybridized with strain of *S. enterica* in the five samples, and the probes Sal1 and Salm-63 were specifically hybridized with *Salmonella* spp. in general. However, different fluorescence signals were observed from the probes indicating different levels of Salmonella spp. contamination. The representative florescence microscopy photomicrographs showing detection of Salmonella species targeted by each oligonucleotide probe are shown in (Fig. 2).

The results of this study have shown the presence of *Salmonella* spp. in all samples using four *Salmonella* specific oligonucleotide probes by employing FISH assay. All of the analyzed samples such as chicken, cutting board, knife, hands and cucumber was found positive for *Salmonella* spp. with different contamination levels. A strong positive hybridization signal with Sapathe3 probe was observed in three samples (Chicken, hands and cucumber). This observation indicates that these three samples were heavily contaminated with *S. enterica* subsp., as this oligonucleotide probe targeted 16S rRNA of *Salmonella enterica* subspp. A closely related study conducted by Zadernowska and Chajecka [8] detected *Salmonella* spp. in food products by FISH method. According to this study, 56 out of 86 food samples were found positive for *Salmonella* using FISH assay. This study suggested that the reason behind a huge number of positive results of *Salmonella* detection by using the FISH method is because this assay seems to be less prone to diverse physical and chemical properties of food products such as temperature, concentration of NaCl, and pH; which can work as stress factors for *Salmonella* spp. Additionally, the chicken samples were observed to have a sufficient number of ribosomes detectable by hybridization with Sal1 and Sal3 probes in comparison to cutting board, knife, hands and cucumber samples. A closely related study by Van asslt et al. [22] evaluated the overall transfer rates of *Campylobacter* for cutting board, knife and hands in the same range as observed in this study.

In this study, no clear correlation was found between the presence of *Salmonella* and the risk of Salmonellosis and this could be due to lack of quantitative data. Nevertheless, the obtained results gave an insight into the overall transfer of *Salmonella*. This indicated that one mistake (e.g. not washing, cutting board) could lead to severe consequences. The fact that transfer of *Salmonella* spp. via various contact surfaces are comparable was also found by Luber et al [12] and this study suggested average transfer of *Campylobacter* from hands or kitchen utensils to ready-to-eat foods ranged from 2.9 -27.5% (moderate contamination). In comparison, in this study, high to moderate level contamination with the *S. enterica* subspp. was observed using two specific probes which targeted this particular *Salmonella* subspecies. The transfer rate of foodborne bacteria (*Salmonella* and *Campylobacter*) from kitchen utensils or hands to ready-to-eat foods such as cucumber slices in this study and in the previous study [12], gave a good indication of the variability of the different surface cross-contamination levels that can be expected in a varied kitchen environment. Three samples (cutting board, knife and cucumber) were found with a low level of *S. enterica* subspp. contamination and this was determined by hybridization of the samples with Sal3 probe using the FISH technique. Furthermore, hybridization with another Salm-63 probe found low levels of *Salmonella* spp. contamination in the three enriched samples (Chicken, cutting board and knife). Luber et al. [12] reported that cross-contamination was most likely to occur via the hands of the cook. Nevertheless, in this study hands were found with low to moderate level contamination as compared to the other samples. Moreover, the behavioral variation among consumers like washing hands, cutting board, and knife, also play a vital role in various levels of contamination. For instance, [5, 16] demonstrated that consumers followed unsafe practices during the preparation of meals which could lead to Salmonellosis and other foodborne outbreaks. In general, the idea of cross-contamination and its possible consequences are unknown to the most of the food handlers. Therefore, this study was designed to indicate the incidence of *Salmonella* spp. cross contamination during the preparation of fresh chicken under various food handling scenarios. The adherence of *Salmonella* on critical surfaces in the kitchen environment such as cutting board, blades of knife, hands and ready to eat food such as cucumber during and after the preparation of chicken was detected by four *Salmonella* species and subspecies specific gene probes employing FISH assay.

The identity of *Salmonella* detected by FISH assay using specific oligonucleotide probes was further confirmed by the growth of *Salmonella* isolates on Hektoen enteric agar (HEA). All *Salmonella* isolates developed characteristic dark green colonies with black center on the HEA. The overall results of this study indicated varied level of *Salmonella* cross-contamination in the items used for the fresh chicken preparation. This finding proved the occurrence of microbial cross-contamination during the fresh chicken preparation. The transfer of *Salmonella* from chicken to items and from items to cucumber provided an overestimation of Salmonellosis. This study demonstrated that contamination occurs frequently through the use of contaminated utensils in preparing other foods. Furthermore, *Salmonella* has potential to spread from chicken samples to the cutting board and other utensils. The consumer behavior in the household or food restaurant kitchen settings is one of the intrinsic factors which could lead to cross-contamination and foodborne illness.

4. Conclusions

This study provided an overall insight about how cross contamination could happen during the preparation of fresh chicken, and the ability of foodborne bacteria to survive on the food contact surfaces and cross contaminate ready to eat food. In conclusion, the results of this study clearly indicated that the raw chicken contaminated with *Salmonella* could cross-contaminate a large number of utensils in the kitchen environment. All of the analyzed samples (chicken, cutting board, knife, hands and cucumber) were found positive for *Salmonella* spp. with different contamination levels. The experimental data obtained in this study clearly suggest that it is extremely difficult to prevent the spread of *Salmonella* spp. during the preparation of raw poultry-based meals. This study recommends that effective measures should be taken to avoid cross-contamination in the kitchen environment. For example, raw and ready to eat food should be handled separately; the same cutting board and chopping knife should not be used for both raw and ready to eat food. Furthermore, hands and utensils that come into contact with raw foodstuffs must be properly washed and sanitized. This study also has found that even after casual rinsing of the cutting board and knife with tap water, a larger number of *Salmonella* cells remain attached to these critical surfaces. In order to minimize the chances of Salmonellosis, good hygiene practices should be followed by food handling personnel. Further studies are recommended on the consumer behavior in the domestic kitchen environment and more specifically to evaluate the extent of accurate sanitary measures practiced by consumers to prevent cross-contamination. In addition, a study on the effect of hygienic measures on the foodborne bacterial cross-contamination in the UAE is highly recommended.

References

[1] Bisha, B. (2009). Fluorescence in situ hybridization-based detection of Salmonella spp. and Listeria monocytogenes in complex food matrices. Iowa State University.

[2] Carrasco, E., Morales-Rueda, A., & García-Gimeno, R. (2012). Cross-contamination and recontamination by Salmonella in foods: A review. Food Research International, 45, 545–556.

[3] Cogan, T., Bloomfield, S., & Humphrey, T. (1999). The effectiveness of hygiene procedures for prevention of cross-contamination from chicken carcases in the domestic kitchen. Letters in Applied Microbiology, 29, 354–358.

[4] Dawson, P., Han, I., Cox, M., Black, C., & Simmons, L. (2007). Residence time and food contact time effects on transfer of Salmonella Typhimurium from tile, wood and carpet: testing the five-second rule. Journal of Applied Microbiology, 102, 945–953.

[5] De Jong, A., Verhoeff-Bakkenes, L., Nauta, M., & De Jonge, R. (2008). Cross-contamination in the kitchen: effect of hygiene measures. Journal of Applied Microbiology,105 ,615–624.

[6] Fravalo, P., Laisney, M. J., Gillard, M. O., Salvat, G., & Chemaly, M. (2009). Campylobacter transfer from naturally contaminated chicken thighs to cutting boards is inversely related to initial load. Journal of food protection, 72(9), 1836-1840.

[7] Humphrey, T., Martin, K., Slader, J., & Durham, K. (2001). Campylobacter spp. in the kitchen: spread and persistence. Journal of Applied Microbiology , 90, 115S-120S

[8] Khan, M., Suryanarayan, P., Ahmed, M. M., Vaswani, R. B., & Faheem, S. M. (2010). Antimicrobial susceptibility of Salmonella isolates from chicken meat samples in Dubai, United Arab Emirates. International Journal of Food, Nutrition and Public Health, 3(2), 149-159.

[9] Kutter S, Hartmann A, Schmid M. 2006. Colonization of barley (Hordeum vulgare) with Salmonella enterica and Listeria spp. FEMS Microbiol Ecol 56: 262-71.

[10] Kyselková, M., Kopecký, J., Frapolli, M., Défago, G., Sagova-Mareckova, M., Grundmann, G. L., & Moënne-Loccoz, Y. (2009). Comparison of rhizobacterial community composition in soil suppressive or conducive to tobacco black root rot disease. The ISME journal, 3(10), 1127.

[11] Luber, P. (2009). Cross-contamination versus undercooking of poultry meat or eggs – which risks need to be managed first. International Journal of Food Microbiology , 134, 21–28

[12] Luber, P., Brynestad, S., Topsch, D., Scherer, K., & Bartelt, E. (2006). Quantification of Campylobacter Species Cross-Contamination during Handling of Contaminated Fresh Chicken Parts in Cross-Contamination during Handling of Contaminated Fresh Chicken Parts in Kitchens. Environ. Microbiol, 72(1):66.

[13] Nzouankeu, A., Ngandjio, A., Ejenguele, G., Njine, T., & Wouafo, M. (2010). Multiple contaminations of chickens with Campylobacter, Escherichia coli and Salmonella in Yaounde (Cameroon). J Infect Dev Ctries, 4(9), 583-586.

[14] Oliveira, M., Blasco, L., Ferrer, S., & Bernardo, F. (2004). Rapid and simultaneous detection of Salmonella spp. and Listeria monocytogenes in milk by Fluorescent In Situ Hybridisation. RPCV, 99 (552) 215-218

[15] Olsen, K.N., Henriksen, M., Bisgaard, M., Nielsen, O.L., Christensen, H., 2008. Investigation of chicken intestinal bacterial communities by 16S rRNA targeted fluorescence in situ hybridization. Antonie van Leeuwenhoek 94, 423–437.

[16] Ravishankar, S., Zhu, L., Jaroni, D. (2010). Assessing the cross contamination and transfer rates of Salmonella enterica. Food Microbiology, 27, 791-794

[17] Redmond, E. C., & Griffith, C. J. (2010). Home food safety and consumer responsibility. Medical and Health Sciences-Volume X, 88.

[18] Reij, M. W., Den Aantrekker, E. D., & ILSI Europe Risk Analysis in Microbiology Task Force. (2004). Recontamination as a source of pathogens in processed foods. International Journal of Food Microbiology, 91(1), 1-11.

[19] Satin, M. (2008). Food alert!: the ultimate sourcebook for food safety. Infobase Publishing.

[20] Soares, V., Pereira, J., Viana, C., Izidoro, T., Bersot, L., & Pinto, J. (2012). Transfer of Salmonella Enteritidis to four types of surfaces after cleaning procedures and cross-contamination to tomatoes. Food Microbiology, 30 , 453-456.

[21] Usha, M., Tunung, R., Chai, L., Ghazali, F., Cheah, Y., Nishibuchi, M., & Son, R. (2010). A study on Campylobacter jejuni cross-contamination during chilled broiler preparation. International Food Research Journal, 17, 107-115

[22] Van Asselt, E., De Jong, A., De Jonge, R., & Nauta, M. (2008). Cross-contamination in the kitchen: estimation of transfer rates for cutting boards, hands and knives. Journal of Applied Microbiology, 105, 1392–1401.

[23] Zadernowska, A., & Chajęcka, W. (2012). Detection of Salmonella spp. presence in food. In Salmonella-A Dangerous Foodborne Pathogen. InTech.

10

Trends of Breastfeeding in the United Arab Emirates (UAE)

Zainab Taha

College of Natural and Health Sciences, Zayed University, Abu Dhabi, U.A.E.

Corresponding Author: Zainab Taha; email: zainab.taha@zu.ac.ae

Abstract

In 1990, the World Health Organization (WHO) and the United Nations Children's Fund (UNICEF) declared a "global goal" for protection, promotion and support of breastfeeding (Innocenti Declaration) (WHO/UNICEF 1990). In 1991, health care authorities in the UAE started to implement breastfeeding promotion and support programs across the country. To date, there are ongoing national efforts and investments in these programs including development and update of policies and strategies. This mini review evaluates the trends of infant and child feeding practices in the UAE over the last few decades to assess the progress attributed to the rollout and implementation of breastfeeding promotion programs. The ongoing journey of promotion of breast feeding has led to an increase of the percentage of infants who were ever breast fed from 60% during the late 1970s to 95% in 2015. There is still a large potential to improve practices; fortunately the progress has been steady and hopefully the desired targets will eventually be achieved.

Keywords: Breastfeeding, Infant feeding, United Arab Emirates

1. Introduction

The numerous benefits of breastfeeding for infants and mothers have long been recognized, understood and well documented. Breastfeeding plays a critical role in the health and development of children and is an essential predictor of infant and child nutrition, health and survival. The WHO recommends exclusive breastfeeding (EBF) during the first six months of life [13]. The WHO defines EBF as offering only breast milk to infants up to six months of age; the exceptions are oral rehydration salts (ORS), nutritional supplements (vitamins & minerals) and medications as needed.

Early and EBF enables children to survive and thrive, it supports healthy brain development, improves cognitive performance and is further associated with better educational achievement at age 5 [22]. In addition, it decreases the hospitalization rates for diarrheal diseases and respiratory tract infections [21]. Furthermore, infants who are exclusively breastfed up to six months are less likely to develop obesity, diabetes and cardiovascular disease later in life [4, 9, 10, 24] (Chung et al., 2007). In addition to EBF from birth to 6 months of age, the WHO also recommends timely initiation of safe, nutritionally-adequate and age-appropriate complementary feeding at six months with continued breastfeeding till the age of two. Continuation of breastfeeding after 6 months of age continues to be critical for the nutrition and growth of the child. (Pan American Health Organization 2001).

Despite the well documented evidence of EBF advantages; its implementation remains to be a global challenge including developed countries [6, 21] (Chung et al., 2007). Sadly, it is even less common in developing countries [11, 14]. In spite of all of the global efforts on promotion of breastfeeding, the UNICEF global databases for 2015 reports that only 38% of children under 6 months of age are exclusively breastfed [22].

2. UAE Background (Breastfeeding Promotion Policies, Programs, and Legislations)

Traditionally breastfeeding has been the customary means of feeding infants since time immemorial. This has been driven by culture, tradition and religion. The UAE is a Muslim country and in Islam breastfeeding is regarded as a prospect of mothers; and women are urged to continue breastfeeding their babies for two years [20]. However, with modernization of life and misconceptions about infant nutrition, feeding practices have gradually deviated from breastfeeding. The UAE is embracing the international recommendations of the WHO and UNICEF on infant and child feeding practices- is promoting breastfeeding as the ideal method of feeding infants and young children. Breastfeeding promotion, protection and support programs have received considerable attention by the UAE Ministry of Health (MOH) and all health care authorities. Various policy initiatives, including the International Code of Marketing of Breast Milk Substitutes (1981), the Innocenti Declaration (1990), the Baby-Friendly Hospital Initiative (BFHI) (1991), and the Global Strategy for Infant and Young Child Feeding (2002) have been developed and adopted by the UAE to improve breastfeeding outcomes. Furthermore, the MOH issued a national infant feeding policy to be implemented throughout the country. The UAE infant feeding policy states that infants should be breast fed exclusively until six months of age [6].

Furthermore, in 2014 the country's Federal National Council passed a draft clause in the child rights law to make breastfeeding mandatory for the first two years of an infant's life [19]. Recently a decree has been issued that extended the 60-day period of paid maternity leave to 90 days. The legislation granted mothers a continuous two hours for breastfeeding every day for the first six months after maternity leave and an hour for the subsequent six months for one year from the day of giving birth as compared to the previous provision of one hour.

The MOH has also encouraged hospitals and health centers with maternity facilities to adopt the "Baby Friendly Initiative". The number of baby friendly hospitals is currently 16 hospitals in addition to 16 primary health care centers. Efforts towards breastfeeding promotion were further extended in 2015 through the declaration of the Sharjah City as the Middle East's first baby-friendly city following the successful adoption of the main standards for this rating.

The experience of the health workforce in Sharjah is extraordinary and should be acknowledged and recommended for further implementation not only by other emirates in the UAE, but also at a broader spectrum; in the Middle East and Gulf region. The main activity in Sharjah comprised a breastfeeding campaign (the Sharjah Baby-Friendly Campaign) which started in 2012. The main components of the campaign included; Baby-Friendly Health Facility, Mother-Friendly Workplace, Breastfeeding-Friendly Nursery, and Mother-Baby Friendly Public Place [1]. The results of the campaign have shown a positive impact on breastfeeding promotion, protection, and support as illustrated by the increased exclusive breastfeeding rate at 6 months from 18.1% in 2011 to 39.86% following the campaign.

3. An Overview of breastfeeding status over the past four decades

Mixed feeding has been the predominant practice for infant nutrition during late 1970s; it was reported that formula, solid and other liquid foods were introduced as early as one month [5]. Breastfeeding was never attempted for 40% of infants and the duration was less than three months for 50% of the mothers who breastfed their babies. A survey conducted by The National Child Health (NHS) in 1988 revealed that 88% of mothers ever breastfed their infants. It also documented a higher rate of breastfeeding in multiparous women as compared to first born infants. The mean duration of breastfeeding was 9.8 months and it was longer in older mothers (12 month for mothers over 40 years old versus 7 months for mothers under 20 years old)

(The National Child Health Survey: UAE, 1988). In 1992 bottle feeding continued to be very dominant, the National Nutrition Survey in the UAE showed that 42% of mothers gave their children bottles during the first month, 21% during the second, and 9% during the third month after birth [17]. The health care authorities in the UAE started to implement a breastfeeding support program following the 1990 Innocenti Declaration. The MOH adopted this program with the key objective of optimal infancy and young child feeding. It encouraged hospitals and health centers with maternity facilities to be baby-friendly hospitals and practice the ten steps to successful breastfeeding. A follow up survey in 1995 showed some improvement with 23% of infants breastfed within an hour of birth and the rate of ever breastfeeding 93 %. However, bottle feeding was still predominant at a percentage of 71.9% [16].

The progress of breastfeeding has been slow despite the ongoing efforts by the health care authorities to influence the infant feeding practices. In 1997, it was reported that 70% of infants in a cohort in the city of Al Ain received non-milk supplements during the first month. Nevertheless, the wheel of change was slowly rolling with 51% of mothers starting breastfeeding on the first day after birth and 4% of infants exclusively breastfed during the first month [2].

The health care authorities continued to conduct studies and surveys to follow the practices of infant feeding and to tailor their policies and support programs accordingly. In 1999, a study in Al Ain reported that 28% of mothers exclusively breastfed their infants and 46% of infants were breastfed for 4-6 months. Inclusion of milk supplements generally occurred early with 76.1% of infants given milk supplements before the end of their first month. Fresh cow and goat milk were the most common supplements [18]. A survey conducted in 2000 showed some progress; 34% of infants were exclusively breastfed to four months of age, 50% of infants were still receiving some breast milk at 12–15 months. The rate of women initiating breastfeeding has increased to 97% with over 50% of them starting within 6 hours after birth (23% within the first hour and 29% within six hours). However, 36% of infants were given infant formula along with breastmilk before 3 months postpartum [7].

A prospective study was conducted in Sharjah in 2006 to investigate breastfeeding patterns at day 1, 1 month, and 6 months postpartum. It showed that the exclusive breastfeeding rate was 76.5% on day 1, 48.4% at 1 month, and 13.3% at 6 months. 16.1% of mothers had stopped breastfeeding by 6 months. It also documented that pethidine use was associated with lower levels of exclusive breastfeeding at 1 month and that maternal education was the most significant determinant of breastfeeding behavior at 6 months [3].

In 2013, a three – city study was conducted in Abu Dhabi, Dubai and Al Ain, to assess the patterns and determinants of breastfeeding and complementary feeding practices. According to the results of this study, almost all the mothers had initiated breastfeeding (98%). The mean duration of breastfeeding was 8.6 months. The percentage of infants who were exclusively breastfed for 4 and 6 months was 7.4% and 1.9% respectively. The majority of the infants (83.5%) in the three cities received solid food before the age of 6 months (Radwan, 2013).

Most recently a study on breastfeeding was conducted in Abu Dhabi and the results showed that early initiation of breastfeeding was 95%. It was very impressive that only 3% infants were exclusively fed infant formula. Almost half of the women in the study breastfed their infant within the first hour after birth and a further 18% initiating breastfeeding within over 4 hours after birth. The majority (61%) of mothers planned to breastfeed for more than 18 months. Only 9% of the mothers in this study intended to stop breastfeeding before their infant was six months of age. However, follow up revealed low rates of exclusive breastfeeding, 5% and 0 % at 3 and 6 months respectively [8].

4. Conclusions

Although the rates of exclusive breastfeeding in the UAE are still suboptimal, the review of the various studies and surveys conducted on breastfeeding indicates steady improvement. However, the results point to some variation which could be attributed to the strong diversity among people living in the UAE. Regardless of these variations, it is evident that the UAE undertook concrete measures towards in supporting, promoting and protecting breastfeeding.

The "Federal National Council" passed a clause in the child rights law to make breastfeeding mandatory for the first two years of an infant's life. Awareness campaigns and support for mothers are continually being made available across the UAE to encourage mothers to exclusively breastfeed for 6 months. The number of baby friendly hospitals in the country is increasing. Besides, the MOH is currently finalizing the "UAE Code of Marketing of Breastmilk Substitutes" which will be implemented to regulate the marketing of breast-milk substitutes, feeding bottles and teats. However, experts in the field may argue that despite the concrete efforts of the UAE in implementing the recommendations of the UNICEF & WHO on supporting, protecting, and promoting breastfeeding, the practices of breastfeeding as measured by the rate of exclusive breastfeeding fall short against the target. This could be attributed to a number of barriers that make it difficult for women to exclusively breastfeed their infants up to the age of 6 months. Such barriers include i) the perception that babies continue to be hungry after breastfeeding due to insufficient milk; ii) maternal health problems; iii) breast pain associated with incorrect positioning; iv) the need to resume work or education; and v) pressure from family members. However, despite the existence of these barriers, the MOH efforts are expected to improve if not resolve them completely, and therefore increase the rate of exclusive breastfeeding.

5. Recommendations

Health providers in the UAE and all organizations and institutions involved in child health and wellbeing should collaborate to support breastfeeding through the following actions:

1. Investment in research to enhance the development of targeted evidence-based strategies for social and behavioural change.
2. Public and professional education to overcome the current barriers to successful exclusive breastfeeding.
3. Reinforcement of policies and systems that enable working mothers to exclusively breastfeed their children up to 6 months of age, through providing mothers with time, space and support
4. Training and supportive supervision to build the capacity of health workers to better counsel and support mothers.
5. Building on the successful model of Al Sharjah, the health workforce in the UAE should work towards national implementation of baby friendly environment.

References

[1] Al Ghazal H, Rashid S, Ruf E. The Sharjah Baby-Friendly Campaign: A Community-Based Model for Breastfeeding Promotion, Protection, and Support. 2015; 10(9):437-441. https://doi.org/10.1089/bfm.2015.0095

[2] Al-Mazroui MJ, Oyejide CO, Bener A, Cheema MY. Breastfeeding and supplemental feeding for neonates in Al-Ain, United Arab Emirates; Journal of Tropical Pediatrics 1997; 43(5):304-306

[3] Al Tajir, G.K.; Sulieman, H.; Badrinath, P. Intragroup differences in risk factors for breastfeeding outcomes in a multicultural community. J Hum Lact 2006; 22:39-47

[4] Arenz S, Ruckerl R, Koletzko B, von Kries R. Breast-feeding and childhood obesity: a systematic review. Int J Obes Relat Metab Disord 2004; 28:1247-1256.

[5] Autret M, Miladi S. Report on the state of food and nutrition in the United Arab Emirates. Part II. UNICEF; 1979

[6] Donath S, Amir LH. Rates of breastfeeding in Australia by State and socio-economic status: Evidence from the 1995 National Health Survey. J Paediatr Child Health 2000; 36:164-168.

[7] Fikri M, Farid S. United Arab Emirates Family Health Survey; United Arab Emirates Ministry of Health: Abu Dhabi, United Arab Emirates, 2000.

[8] Gardner H, Green K, Gardner A. Infant Feeding Practices of Emirati Women in the Rapidly Developing City of Abu Dhabi, United Arab Emirates. Int J Environ Res Public Health 2015; 12:10923-10940.

[9] Gillman MW. The first months of life: a critical period for development of obesity. AJCN 2008; 87(6):1587-1589.

[10] Horta BL, Bahln R, Martines JC, Victora CG. Evidence on the long- term effects of breastfeeding: systematic reviews and meta-analyses. Geneva: WHO; 2007; 52-57.

[11] Imdad A, Yakoob MY, Bhutta ZA. Effect of breastfeeding promotion interventions on breastfeeding rates, with special focus on developing countries. BMC Public Health 2011; 11 (Suppl. 3). doi:10.1186/1471-2458-11-S3-S24.

[12] Innocenti Declaration on the Protection, Promotion and Support of Breastfeeding. Florence, Italy, WHO/UNICEF (Spedale degli Innocenti), 1990.

[13] Kramer MS and Ritsuko K. The Optimal Duration of Exclusive Breastfeeding: A Systematic Review: World Health Organization, 2002.

[14] Lauer JA, Betrán AP, Victora CG, de Onís M, Barros AJ. Breastfeeding patterns and exposure to suboptimal breastfeeding among children in developing countries: Review and analysis of nationally representative surveys. BMC Med 2004; 2. doi:10.1186/1741-7015-2-26.

[15] Ministry of Health UAE: The National Child Health survey, UAE Ministry of Health. UAE, 1988.

[16] National Family Health Survey, Ministry of Health.1995.

[17] National Nutrition Survey: UAE Ministry of Health. UAE, 1992.

[18] Osman NA, El-Sabban FF. Infant feeding practices in Al-Ain, United Arab Emirates. East Mediterr. Health J 1999; 5:103-110.

[19] Salem O. FNC passes mandatory breastfeeding clause for Child Rights law. In The National; Abu Dhabi Media: Abu Dhabi, United Arab Emirates, 2014.

[20] Shaikh U, Ahmed O. Islam and infant feeding. Breastfeed Med 2006; 1:164-167

[21] Quigley MA, Kelly YJ, Sacker A. Breastfeeding and hospitalization for diarrheal and respiratory infection in the United Kingdom Millennium cohort study. Pediatrics 2007; 119:e837-e842.

[22] UNICEF, WHO. Breastfeeding Advocacy Initiative: For the Best Start in Life. Advocacy Strategy. 2015.

[23] World Health Organization (WHO): Indicators for assessing infant and young child feeding practices Part 1 Definitions. Geneva: WHO, 2008.

[24] WHO: Global Strategy for Infant and Young Child Feeding. Geneva: WHO, 2003.

Intradialytic Aerobic Exercise in the United Arab Emirates: A Descriptive Study

Nada Salhab[1], Mirey Karavetian[2], Jeroen Kooman[3], and Enrico Fiaccadori[4]

[1]Maastricht University, Minderbroedersberg 4-6, 6211 LK Maastricht, The Netherlands
[2]Zayed University, Academic City – Dubai, United Arab Emirates
[3]University Hospital Maastricht, P. Debyelaan 25, 6229 HX Maastricht, The Netherlands
[4]Parma University, Via Università, 12, 43121 Parma PR, Italy

Corresponding Author: Nada Salhab; email: n.salhab@maastricht university.nl

Abstract

Aim. Intradialytic exercise (IDE) improves hyperphosphatemia management in hemodialysis (HD) patient in addition to other clinical outcomes. The aim of the study is to present the strategies needed to integrate such a protocol in an HD unit in UAE and patients' baseline characteristics. **Methods.** The largest HD unit in Sharjah emirate was chosen. All eligible patients (n = 57) in the unit were included. Patients were stable adults HD patients who served as their own controls. The intervention included an aerobic low intensity IDE of 45 minutes per HD session, tailored to each patient's fitness scale (BORG scale) for 6 months. Patients were educated on the importance of exercise. Outcome measures were barriers to exercise, serum phosphorus (P), urea reduction ratio (URR), malnutrition inflammation score, quality of life (QOL using euroqol5) collected at baseline and post intervention. **Results.** A total of 41 patients completed the study, 61% were males and 90.2%, 53.7% and 14.6% suffered from hypertension, diabetes and cardiovascular disease, respectively. Hyperphosphatemia was prevalent among 75% of the patients with a mean of 5.76 ± 1.66 mg/dl. The mean age was 48 ± 14.37 years, BMI 24.98 ± 6.09 kg/m^2, URR 71.88 ± 8.52%, and Kt/v 1.32 ± 1.09. The main barrier to exercise was identified to be fatigue on HD days by 58.5% of patients, followed by fear of getting hurt (36.6%). Finally, 80.4% of patients were mildly malnourished and QOL scale was 65.02% ± 18.54. **Conclusion.** Our study highlighted the widespread of hyperphosphatemia and malnutrition in our sample. The IDE regimen, if proven effective in future studies, could be integrated in the routine practice and may improve patients' outcomes.

Keywords: hemodialysis, exercise, quality of life, phosphorus, urea

1. Introduction

Chronic kidney disease (CKD) has been recently recognized as a global health concern [1] with a prevalence of 13.4% worldwide [2]. CKD poses an increased mortality rate compared to their age-matched healthy population [3]. In the United Arab Emirates (UAE), the estimated total number of dialysis patients in 2014 was 1870, out of which 94% are on hemodialysis (HD), with a prevalence rate of 210 per million population [4].

Hyperphosphatemia, defined as high serum phosphorus level, is highly prevalent among HD patients and a known risk factor for mortality [5]. The Kidney Disease Improving Global Outcomes (KDIGO) 2017 guidelines recommend lowering the phosphate levels toward the normal range; hyperphosphatemia management includes dialysis, limiting dietary phosphate intake, and the usage of phosphate binder, while restricting the dose of calcium-based phosphate binders [6]. It is documented that a weekly dialysis of more than 30 hours is required for a complete clearance of serum phosphate (P) without the use of P-binders [7]; yet, in the UAE, the reality remains that HD sessions in routine practice accumulate to a maximum of 12 hours per week [8]. Poor serum P control due to high P-to-protein ratio can pose the risk of malnutrition on HD patients, a phenomenon common among these patients [9]. Furthermore, sedentary lifestyle is widespread in HD patients, and stage 4 and 5 CKD cases report to have the lowest physical activity (PA) levels [10]. This is despite the fact that the literature is clear on the positive effect of PA on the management of hyperphosphatemia [11], and the negative effect of low PA on quality of life (QOL) [12] and nutritional status [13]. Broers et al. were able to demonstrate a positive correlation between the QOL-physical component and nutritional indices [13]. Thus, finding an adjunctive therapy to facilitate hyperphosphatemia management and increase PA levels becomes crucial.

Intradialytic exercise (IDE) has shown to ameliorate solute clearance by increasing blood flow and thus hyperphosphatemia management of HD [14]. Patients trained on a cycle ergometer for 20–30 minutes during the first 2 hours of HD increased their phosphate removal [11] and improved their QOL—physical component [15] and their QOL total score [16]. IDE had a positive effect on dialysis efficiency, specifically on Kt/v [17] and the urea reduction ratio (URR) [18]. In addition, IDE showed a non-significant decrease in hospitalization rate [19].

For IDE to be a routine procedure for HD patients, an HD unit needs proper exercise equipment, optimal exercise strategies tailored to the patients, trained staff and policies [20]. The fact remains that intradialytic training programs are not yet integrated in routine practice worldwide; UAE is not an exception. The feasibility analysis of an IDE program in a developing country is needed, since most of the proof of the efficacy of IDE in HD patients comes from the developed Western countries.

The aim of the current study is to present the study design and protocol of an aerobic exercise program that will be conducted on HD patients in a selected center in the UAE; another aim is to describe the baseline characteristics of the participants regarding the selected outcome parameters: adequacy of dialysis, serum phosphorus, quality of life, exercise behavior, barriers to exercise, and malnutrition inflammation score.

2. Methods

2.1. Study design

A quasi-experimental intervention with pre- and post-evaluation design was planned in Al Qassimi hospital's HD unit in Sharjah, UAE. This study was conducted according to the Helsinki Ethical Declaration of 1975 as revised in 1983 and received ethical approval from the Research Ethics Committee of the Ministry of Health and Prevention of UAE (MOHP/DXB/SUBC/NO-5/2016) and that of Zayed University (ZU15_118_F). The study was registered in the ClinicalTrials.gov (ID: NCT03131804). Patients were informed of the study protocol, its risks and benefits, confidentiality, the need for the study team to go through their medical files, and their ability to voluntarily enter and exit the study. The actual patient's name list was maintained with the primary investigator (PI), numerical identification was used instead of names to ensure confidentiality and anonymity. Moreover, the filled and signed consent forms and questionnaires were kept with the PI in a locked drawer.

2.2. Study methodology

Convenient sample technique was used; all patients in the chosen HD unit, who were eligible, that is, satisfy the pre-set inclusion criteria and consented, were included in the intervention, resulting in a convenient sampling. Inclusion criteria were stable adult HD patients, on HD for ≥ 3 months, free of acute diseases and specific cardiovascular problems (cardiac pacemaker, uncontrolled blood pressure, symptomatic ischemic heart disease, arrhythmias, deep vein thrombosis, severe dyspnea), of either gender, not practicing an exercise program at the time of the study, capable to communicate, fully aware of the study protocol, able to perform the cycle peddler and provided a consent form. Exclusion criteria were patients not meeting the inclusion criteria; in addition to any of the following: dialyzed from a femoral fistula, suffering from severe anemia (hemoglobin: < 9g/dl) [21] and/or uncontrolled diabetes.

Five research assistants (RAs) were recruited to conduct the study. They were trained by the PI on study protocol and data collection tools. A licensed physiotherapist of the selected hospital was consulted for the planning of the exercise program, choosing the proper static bicycle and for ongoing supervision of the exercise program.

2.3. Sample size

The outcome was the decrease in serum phosphate. Power analysis was conducted using the GPower 3.1 software (GPower 3.1) (Retrieved from `https://www.campbellcollaboration.org/escalc/html/EffectSizeCalculator-SMD1.php`. (accessed January 15, 2017).), based on the effect size (d = |0.56|) retrieved from [22], an RCT conducted in Iran. The sample size yielded by the power analysis (n = 34), which was inflated by 72.7% to account for drop out, leading to a total included sample of 57. We approached all eligible patients (n = 57) out of which 41 consented and were included in the analysis.

2.4. Conduct of Study

The study is designed according to three phases: baseline (T_0), intervention (T_1) and follow-up (T_2).

Phase 1: Baseline (T_0) with 2 months duration. The RAs validated the questionnaires, conducted a 2-weeks pilot study on 10 HD patients (results of which were later discarded), and completed the baseline assessment for all consented patients. Furthermore, eligible patients were educated on the importance of exercise, specifically IDE, to their health prior to the start of the study by the PI. Finally, patients were assessed using the study outcome measures and data were recorded.

Phase 2: Intervention (T_1) with 6 months duration. The RAs and the physiotherapist implemented the aerobic IDE using a static cycle peddler parallel to an ongoing monthly education on the importance of exercise and on how to integrate it in regular life. The RAs trained the patients on the exercise program and recorded the intensity (using the Borg scale) (Centers for Disease Control and Prevention) [23] and the duration of the exercise for each patient as well as the patient's complaints and reasons for dropout, if any. In addition, the blood pressure and pulse rate were taken at the beginning of the exercise and at every 15-minutes interval. Exercise were not initiated or stopped if the blood pressure was above 200/110 based on the recommendation from the literature [15]. The exercise program consists of cycling on a static bicycle "Pedal Exerciser KD" for 45 minutes during the first 2 hours of dialysis to avoid stress in the second half of the HD session; the peddler was positioned and stabilized in front of the patients, while they lied in their dialysis bed. The exercise modality is as follows: A 2-minutes warm-up cycling at the lowest resistance of the cycle ergometer [24]; thereafter, the conditioning phase consisted of cycling at patient's preferred resistance, while advising the patient to adjust the intensity to achieve moderate intensity exercise; exercise intensity was assessed using the Borg scale of perceived exertion and patients were encouraged to reach an average exertion score of 12. The study at all times was under the direct supervision of a nephrologist and physiotherapist assigned to the study by the hospital; in case of any discomfort, the intervention was stopped immediately. As a motivational tool, the patient's activity level (number of minutes exercised) was recorded on a tracking chart posted in the unit, and the patient with the highest performance was rewarded at the end of the intervention. At the end of this phase, patients were evaluated using all the study parameters.

Phase 3: Follow-up (T_2), 3 months post intervention. During this phase, there was no interaction between patients and the research team, and at the end, patients were re-evaluated on all study parameters.

2.5. Data collection

Data was collected utilizing validated questionnaires and blood tests from patient hospital charts (Table 1). All questionnaires that were originally not in Arabic (Barriers to Exercise and QOL) were translated to Arabic (local language), prior to the study by two translators whose first language was Arabic. Afterwards, each questionnaire was re-translated to English by a dietitian whose first language was English and who also knew Arabic. The questionnaires were administered by the recruited RAs at three points in time: T_0, T_1 and T_2. For quality control purposes, two questionnaires were administered at a time and reviewed prior to administering the next.

3. Outcome Measures

3.1. Objective tools

Data from the medical chart of each HD patient was collected that included demographics, biochemical markers [Serum Phosphorus (P) mg/dl, Parathyroid Hormone (PTH) pmol/L, Calcium Phosphorus Product (Ca x P) mg^2/dl^2, Hemoglobin (HGB) g/dl, Kt/v, and Urea Reduction Ratio (URR) %]. Demographics were collected only at $T_0$and the remaining information from patient file was collected at T_0 (average of 3 months prior to study), and further at T_1 (monthly throughout the study) and T_2 (average of 3 months post intervention).

3.2. Subjective tools

Four questionnaires were used in this study. All of which were administered at three phases of the study. RAs helped patients fill the questionnaires.

1. Malnutrition Inflammation Score (MIS) adapted from Kalantar-Zadeh et al. [25] had 10 components, each with four levels of severity from 0 (normal) to 3 (severely abnormal). The sum of all 10 MIS components ranged from 0 (normal) to 30 (severely abnormal); a higher score reflected severe degree of malnutrition and inflammation.
2. Exercise behavior, attitude and knowledge questionnaire were developed by the authors of this study. They included seven questions, each with multiple answers to choose from (See Appendix 1, Supplemental Material 1).
3. Barriers to physical activity questionnaire adapted from Fiaccadori et al. [26] included 24 questions that evaluated barriers to physical activity (psychological, physical, and economical barriers) in addition to the lack of time factor.
4. Quality of life was measured using QOL "EQ-5D-5L" questionnaire [27]. It assessed five health concepts: mobility, self-care, usual activities, pain/discomfort, and anxiety/depression. Each question had five answer choices. In addition, patients marked their self-rated health on a visual scale from 0–100.

3.3. Statistical analysis

Data was analyzed using the Statistical Package for the Social Sciences (SPSS version 21). Results were considered statistically significant at $P < 0.05$ to guarantee 95% confidence interval. Descriptive data was conducted, categorical data were reported as frequencies and percentages counts; normality was checked for all continuous variables and statistical analyses were conducted accordingly (bivariate analysis). In order to keep the tables homogenous, means, SD, min. and max. were kept on. Moreover, median and interquartile range values were presented for all continuous variables.

4. Results

A total of 41 patients met the inclusion criteria and consented out of the 150 patients dialyzing in the selected HD unit (Figure 1).

4.1. Baseline sample characteristics

A descriptive analysis of baseline data (Tables 1 and 2) showed that 61% of the population was male with a mean age of 48.0 and mean BMI 24.98 kg/m^2. The majority of the patients were married (78.0%) and were Arab (Emirati and non-Emirati; 75.6%). More than half of the patients

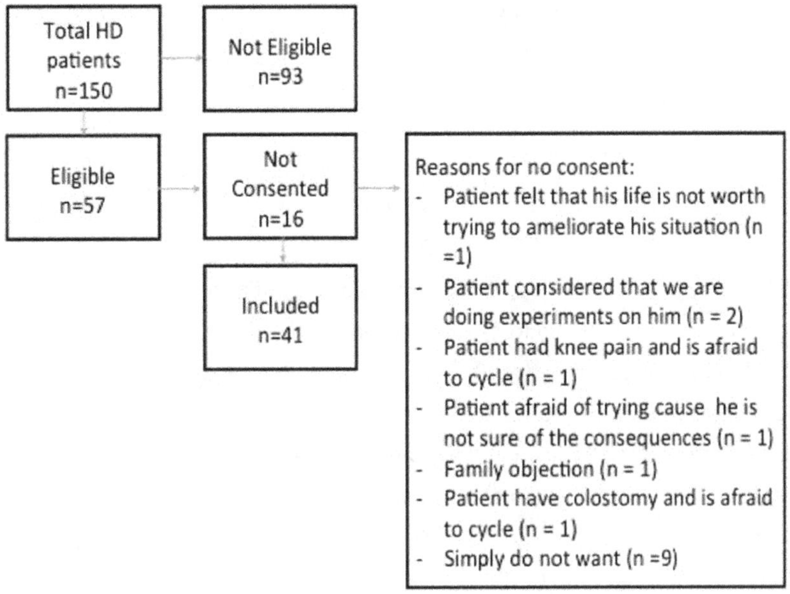

Figure 1: Flow diagram of the patients.

did not work (58.5%) and 43.9% had university degrees. Diabetes was the most common primary cause of HD initiation (56.1%), followed by hypertension (22%). The most common comorbidities included hypertension (90.2%), followed by diabetes (53.7%). Mean of recorded blood parameters were as follows: serum phosphorus (5.76 mg/dl), calcium and phosphorus byproduct (48.67 mg^2/dl^2), PTH (54.28 pmol/L), hemoglobin (10.72 g/dl), Kt/v (1.32), and URR (71.88%).

Perceived barriers to exercise among the study participants (Table 4) revealed only 1 patient (2.4%) reporting no barriers at all, followed by 14.6% of them reporting 1 barrier, 36.6% had 2–4 barriers, 36.6% had 5–9 barriers, 9.8% had 10 or more barriers. The most frequently reported barriers were fatigue on dialysis days (58.5%), fear of getting hurt (36.6%), and fatigue on non-dialysis days (34.1%).

The mean of self-rated QOL visual analogue scale was 65.02 ±18.54 (min: 25; max: 100). As for the rest of the QOL domains (Table 5), almost half of the patients did not have any problem in walking (48.8%), and most of them were independent in their routine daily self-care (90%) and activities (68.3%). Pain and discomfort were reported by 9.8% of the patients and anxiety and depression by 7.3%.

5. Discussion

The current study is the first of its kind in UAE to assess the effect of IDE on clinical, behavioral, nutritional and quality of life outcomes among HD patients. We were able to reveal patient characteristics on all study parameters.

	n (%)		n (%)
Gender, Male	25 (61)	Primary Cause of Hemodialysis	
		Diabetes	23 (56.1)
		Hypertension	9 (22)
		Nephritis	5 (12.2)
		Others	4 (9.8)
Nationality		Hemodialysis Initiation	
Emirati	8 (19.5)	<1 year	12 (29.3)
Non-Emirati - Arab	23 (56.1)	1-4 years	15 (36.6)
Non-Emirati - Other	10 (24.4)	>4 years	14 (34.1)
Social Status		Comorbidities*	
Single	8 (19.5)	Diabetes	22 (53.7)
Married	32 (78)	Hypertension	37 (90.2)
Other	1 (2.4)	Cardiovascular Disease	6 (14.6)
		Others	13 (31.7)
Work, No	24 (58.5)	Hyperphosphatemia (Serum P >4.6 mg/dl)	31 (75)[¥]
Education Level			
Illiterate	4 (9.8)		
Read and Write	4 (9.8)		
Elementary	5 (12.2)		
High School	10 (24.4)		
University	18 (43.9)		

TABLE 1: Baseline characteristics of patients (categorical data) (n = 41).

While existing studies in the region are limited to their descriptive and cross-sectional nature [28, 29], or to their short intervention time [30], the current study is unique in its prospective interventional design implementing the IDE program in UAE.

The study sample was similar to the general HD population in the Gulf countries and UAE in particular in many socio-demographic and clinical aspects. Our ethnic and culturally diversified sample is reflective of the nature of the UAE population [31]. Moreover, our participants were relatively young, and more than half were male. This male predominance in the HD population is a global finding [32] and is consistent with "The Dialysis Outcomes and Practice Patterns Study" (DOPPS) results reported on patients in Gulf countries in general and specifically in the UAE [4]. As for the reasons for initiation of HD, diabetes and hypertension were the most common causes in our sample; a similar finding was reported from DOPPS [4]. Finally, hypertension as a comorbidity was prevalent in more than 90% of the patients in both our sample and the representative sample of DOPPS UAE [4]. Moreover, more than half of the patients did not work and 43.9% had university degrees; the former figure is comparable to DOPPS results where

	Normal Values	Mean ± SD	Min/Max	Median	IQR
Age (years)		48.00 ± 14.37	20/74	50.00	36.50-58.00
BMI (kg/m^2)	20-25	24.98 ± 6.09	17.06/46.14	23.32	21.26-26.70
URR (%)	≥ 65	71.88 ± 8.52	50.79/89.62	71.69	66.14-77.23
Kt/v	1.2-1.4	1.32 ± 1.09	1.08/1.63	1.30	1.24-1.37
P (mg/dl)	2.5-4.5	5.76 ± 1.66	1.83/9.32	5.61	4.82-6.48
Ca x P (mg^2/dl^2)	≤ 55	48.67 ± 14.30	15.44/82.86	45.65	39.11-56.65
PTH (pmol/L)	15.90-31.81	54.28 ± 45.60	8.90 /243.2	44.50	24.40-69.30
HGB (g/dl)	13-17	10.72 ± 1.44	7.53/14.1	10.6	9.86-11.56
MIS	0	7.41 ± 3.06	3/17	7.00	5.00-9.00

Note: SD: standard deviation; Min: minimum; Max: maximum; BMI: Body Mass Index; URR: Urea Reduction Ratio; P: Phosphorus; Ca*P: Calcium Phosphorus byproduct; PTH: Parathyroid Hormone; HGB: Hemoglobin; MIS: Malnutrition-Inflammation Score; IQR: Interquartile range.

MIS Scoring System: The total MIS ranges between 0 and 30: 0: normal; 1-10: mildly malnourished; 11-20: moderately malnourished; 21-30: severely malnourished.

Behavior, attitude and knowledge of HD patients regarding exercise are detailed in Table 3. Around one-third of the participants reported at baseline that they did not exercise (31.7%), and more than half of the sample (58.6%) intended to start exercising after consulting their physician. The majority of the patients (92.5 %) perceived exercise as important. Around half of the patient knew that exercise is safe (55%) and were knowledgeable about its health benefits (43.9%).

TABLE 2: Baseline characteristics of patients (continuous data) (n = 41).

62% of HD population in the UAE were unemployed [4], and the latter one is comparable to Dubai Statistic Center results, where 74.1% of the unemployed citizens had university degrees [33]. All these factors allow us to generalize our findings to the general UAE HD population.

Hyperphosphatemia was highly prevalent in our sample at baseline (75%), a number that was far higher than the 38% reported in the DOPPS-UAE [29], but this can be explained by the fact that the latter results were of data collected in 2013, using a cut-off point for hyperphosphatemia as 6mg/dl. The current study followed the KDIGO 2017 guidelines using tight serum P control (> 4.6mg/dl) [6]. Data from other studies, using 5.5mg/dl cut-off point showed around 40% prevalence of hyperphosphatemia in the region [34] and worldwide [35]. Given the high clinical [36] and financial burden of hyperphosphatemia [37] and its management through phosphate binders and specifically non-calcium phosphate binders [38], finding an effective and inexpensive novel means to manage hyperphosphatemia is a necessity in modern nephrology care [39].

The majority of our sample was mildly malnourished (80.4%). This is in line with previous literature, where malnutrition was common among HD patients globally [40] and regionally [41]. In the previous literature, exercise appeared to improve protein energy wasting [42] and thus malnutrition.

		n (%)
Exercise Behavior	Frequency of Exercise per Week	
	Don't exercise	13 (31.7)
	Exercise 1–2 time per week	1 (26.8)
	Exercise 3 or more times per week	17 (41.5)
	Duration of Exercise (among patients who reported exercising once or more)	
	Less than 30 minutes each time	9 (32.1)
	30–40 minutes each time	8 (28.6)
	40 minutes and more each time	11 (29.3)
	Exercise Modality*¥ (among patients who reported exercising once or more)	
	Walking	26 (96.3)
	Jogging /Dancing/Aerobics/Others	4 (14.8)
	Weight training	2 (7.4)
Attitude to Exercise	Intent to Start Exercise	
	After consulting the doctor	24 (58.6)
	Does not know	17 (41.5)
	Attitude toward Exercise Importance on Health¥	
	Important	37 (92.5)
	Not important	3 (7.5)
Knowledge on Exercise	Knowledge about Exercise Safety¥	
	Correct knowledge	22 (55.0)
	False knowledge	18 (45.0)
	Knowledge about the Benefits of Exercise for Hemodialysis Patients*¥	
	Correct knowledge	18 (43.9)
	No knowledge	23 (56.1)

Note: *Percentages do not sum up due to multiple possible answers; ¥Valid percentages are reported.

TABLE 3: Exercise behavior, attitude and knowledge questionnaire.

Despite the positive attitude of our sample about the importance of exercise, time allocated for the physical activity was limited, and walking was almost the only form of exercise performed. These practices are similar to those noted in Delgado and Johansen [43]. This is in line with the sedentarism prevalent among HD patients [10]. This might be attributed to the widespread lack of knowledge among these patients or to the fact that exercise is not routinely advocated by the nephrologist within HD patient management [44]. To date, there are no clear guidelines in the KDIGO or the Kidney Disease Outcomes Quality Initiative (KDOQI) [45] on IDE intensity, modality, and duration.

Barriers	n (%)
Fatigue on dialysis days	24 (58.5)
Fear of getting hurt	15 (36.6)
Fatigue on non-dialysis days	14 (34.1)
Shortness of breath	12 (29.3)
Too many medical problems	11 (26.8)
Chest pain	11 (26.8)
Feelings of helplessness	10 (24.4)
Pain on dialysis days	9 (22.0)
Ulcers on legs and feet	9 (22.0)
Sadness	9 (22.0)
Inability to travel	9 (22.0)
Pain on non-dialysis days	8 (19.5)
Lack of time on dialysis days	8 (19.5)
Can't afford to exercise	8 (19.5)
Lack of safe place for exercise	6 (14.6)
Physician concern	5 (12.2)
No exercise partner	5 (12.2)
I don't want to	5 (12.2)
Family concern	5 (12.2)
Lack of time on non-dialysis days	4 (9.8)
Lack of time because of too many medical appointments	4 (9.8)
No place to exercise	3 (7.3)
Feeling too old	2 (4.9)
Not wanting to be seen doing exercise	1 (2.4)

TABLE 4: Perceived barriers to physical activity.

	No problem n (%)	Slight problem n (%)	Moderate problem n (%)	Severe problem n (%)	Unable / very severe n (%)
Self-care	37 (90.2)	1 (2.4)	1 (2.4)	1 (2.4)	1 (2.4)[a]
Daily Activities	28 (68.3)	2 (4.9)	6 (14.6)	2 (4.9)	3 (7.3)[a]
Anxiety/Depression	24 (58.4)	6 (14.6)	5 (12.2)	3 (7.3)	3 (7.3)[a]
Mobility	20 (48.8)	9 (22)	4 (9.8)	5 (12.2)	3 (7.3)[b]
Pain/Discomfort	17 (41.5)	10 (24.4)	4 (9.8)	6 (14.6)	4 (9.8)[b]
Note: [a]= unable; [b]= very severe					

TABLE 5: EuroQOL 5D-5 L questionnaire.

Most of our patients reported the existence of at least one barrier, 73% had more than two barriers and the most common barrier was "fatigue on dialysis days"; this was in line with other studies [26, 43]. The second most prevalent barrier in our sample was "fear of getting hurt", and very few stated, "I do not want to" for exercise; these findings were unique for our patients and different from the literature [26, 43]. Barriers related to physical limitations and fears surrounding exercise ranked higher than logistics-related barriers in our sample.

The QOL visual analogue scale (VAS) was 65.02 ± 18.54, which was slightly higher than VAS results reported from other countries [46]. Also, the percentage of patients reporting no problem across the five dimensions of EQ-5D-5L was higher than the score reported in another countries [46]. Those differences might be attributed to cultural variances. In fact, while conducting the EuroQOL-5D questionnaire, the research team faced a limitation that was most prevalent in the VAS question, which raised the question of its cultural appropriateness and its suitability to assess the quality of life in this population. Patients showed strong religious beliefs and interpreted sickness as "fate" and the "will of God". When asked to rate their health, many of our patients used the word "Thank God" which was difficult to score. This answer was translated to a high score on the scale. Such impact of religious beliefs influencing the QOL assessment among the chronically ill has been previously reported among other cultures as well [42]. Further validation of the instrument in religious-oriented cultures is recommended.

6. Conclusion

Our baseline findings revealed the hyperphosphatemics and malnourished patients and the barriers impeding them from integrating exercise in their lifestyle. Our results may shed light on this overlooked population and enlighten other researchers and stakeholders about the current situation of hemodialysis patients in the UAE. Furthermore, it will highlight the strategies needed to tailor-made exercise program for HD patients in the UAE.

7. Conflict of Interest

None declared

8. Acknowledgment

The project was under the supervision of Dr Harith Muthana, consultant nephrologist at Al Qassimi Hospital. Dr Muthana assigned a nephrologist for the daily supervision of the research. The physiotherapy department at Al Qassimi Hospital assigned a physiotherapist to help in the exercise program implementation. The College of Natural and Health Sciences department at Zayed University in Dubai and Sharjah campuses provided students who helped us in data collection. Special thanks to the staff and patients in participating in the dialysis unit for facilitating the process.

9. Funding

The study was funded by Zayed University, Dubai, UAE [Research Grant Activity: R16115].

References

[1] K. U. Eckardt, J. Coresh, O. Devuyst, R. J. Johnson, A. Kottgen, A. S. Levey, et al. (2013). Evolving importance of kidney disease: From subspecialty to global health burden. Lancet, 382(9887), 158-169. doi:10.1016/s0140-6736(13)60439-0

[2] N. R. Hill, S. T. Fatoba, J. L. Oke, J. A. Hirst, C. A. O'Callaghan, D. S. Lasserson, et al. (2016). Global prevalence of chronic kidney disease: A systematic review and meta-analysis. PLoS One, 11(7), e0158765. doi:10.1371/journal.pone.0158765

[3] K. L. Johansen, G. M. Chertow, A. V. Ng, K. Mulligan, S. Carey, P.Y. Schoenfeld, et al. (2000). Physical activity levels in patients on hemodialysis and healthy sedentary controls. Kidney International, 57, 2564-2570. doi:10.1046/j.1523-1755.2000.00116.x

[4] A. AlSahow, M. AlRukhaimi, J. A. Wakeel, S. M. G. Al-Ghamdi, S. AlGhareeb, F. Al-Ali, et al. (2016). Demographics and key clinical characteristics of hemodialysis patients from the gulf cooperation council countries enrolled in the dialysis outcomes and practice patters study phase 5 (2012-2015). Saudi Journal of Kidney Diseases Transplantation. 27(6suppl 1), S12-S23.

[5] M. K. Kuhlmann. (2006). Management of hyperphosphatemia. Hemodialysis International, 10(4), 338-345. doi:10.1111/j.1542-4758.2006.00126.x

[6] M. Ketteler, G. A. Block, P. Evenepoel, M. Fukagawa, C. A. Herzog, L. McCann, et al. (2017). Executive summary of the 2017 KDIGO Chronic Kidney Disease-Mineral and Bone Disorder (CKD-MBD) Guideline Update: What's changed and why it matters. Kidney International, 92(1), 26-36. doi:10.1016/j.kint.2017.04.006

[7] C. M. Kjellstrand, T. S. Ing, P. T. Kjellstrand, Odar-Cederlof, I., & Lagg, C. R. (2011). Phosphorus dynamics during hemodialysis. Hemodialysis International, 15(2), 226-233. doi:10.1111/j.1542-4758.2011.00538.x

[8] DOPPS Practice Monitor, Gulf Cooperation Council. Dialysis prescription and dose. March 2017. Retrieved from http://www.dopps.org/DPM/GCC/ (accessed September 13, 2017).

[9] A. M. Mathewson, D. Fouque and A. J. Toft. (2010). Dietary phosphate assessment in dialysis patients. J Renal Nutrition, 20(6), 351-358. doi:10.1053/j.jrn.2010.05.014

[10] D. M. Zelle, G. Klaassen, E. van Adrichem, S. J. Bakker, E. Corpeleijn and G. Navis. (2017). Physical inactivity: A risk factor and target for intervention in renal care. Nature Reviews Nephrology, 13(3), 152-168. doi:10.1038/nrneph.2016.187

[11] A. S. Musavian, A. Soleimani, N. Masoudi Alavi, A. Baseri and F Savari. (2015). Comparing the effects of active and passive intradialytic pedaling exercises on dialysis efficacy, electrolytes, hemoglobin, hematocrit, blood pressure and health-related quality of life. Nursing and Midwifery Studies, 4(1), e25922.

[12] A. A. Lopes, B. Lantz, H. Morgenstern, M. Wang, B. A. Bieber, B. W. Gillespie, et al. (2014). Associations of self-reported physical activity types and levels with quality of life, depression symptoms, and mortality in hemodialysis patients: the DOPPS. Clinical Journal of the American Society of Nephrology, 9(10), 1702-1712. doi:10.2215/cjn.12371213

[13] N. J. Broers, L. A. Usvyat, J. P. Kooman, F. M. van der Sande, E. Lacson, Jr., P. Kotanko, et al. (2015). Quality of life in dialysis patients: A retrospective cohort study. Nephron, 130(2), 105-112. doi:10.1159/000430814

[14] K. Sheng, P. Zhang, L. Chen, J. Cheng, C. Wu and J. Chen. (2014). Intradialytic exercise in hemodialysis patients: A systematic review and meta-analysis. American Journal of Nephrology, 40(5), 478-490. doi:10.1159/000368722

[15] M. C. de Lima, L. Cicotoste Cde, S. Cardoso Kda, L. A. Forgiarini, Jr., M. B. Monteiro, and A. S. Dias. (2013). Effect of exercise performed during hemodialysis: Strength versus aerobic. Renal Failure, 35(5), 697-704. doi:10.3109/0886022x.2013.780977

[16] Y. Wu, Q. He, X. Yin, Q. He, S. Cao and G Ying. (2014). Effect of individualized exercise during maintenance haemodialysis on exercise capacity and health-related quality of life in patients with uraemia. Journal of International Medical Research, 42(3), 718-727. doi:10.1177/0300060513509037

[17] C. Groussard, M. Rouchon-Isnard, C. Coutard, F. Romain, L. Malarde, S. Lemoine-Morel, et al. (2015). Beneficial effects of an intradialytic cycling training program in patients with end-stage kidney disease. Applied Physiology, Nutrition, & Metabolism = Physiologie Appliquee, Nutrition et Metabolisme, 40(6), 550-556. doi:10.1139/apnm-2014-0357

[18] M. De Moura Reboredo, D. M. N. Henrique, R. De Souza Faria, A. Chaoubah, M. G. Bastos and R. B. De Paula. (2010). Exercise training during hemodialysis reduces blood pressure and increases physical functioning and quality of life. Artificial Organs, 34(7), 586-593. doi:10.1111/j.1525-1594.2009.00929.x

[19] K. Parker, X. Zhang, A. Lewin and J. M. MacRae. (2015). The association between intradialytic exercise and hospital usage among hemodialysis patients. Applied Physiology, Nutrition, & Metabolism = Physiologie Appliquee, Nutrition et Metabolisme, 40(4), 371-378. doi:10.1139/apnm-2014-0326

[20] K. Parker. (2016). Intradialytic exercise is medicine for hemodialysis patients. Current Sports Medicine Reports, 15(4), 269-275. doi:10.1249/jsr.0000000000000280

[21] A. S. Kliger, R. N. Foley, D. S. Goldfarb, S. L. Goldstein, K. Johansen, A. Singh, et al. (2013). KDOQI US commentary on the 2012 KDIGO Clinical Practice Guideline for Anemia in CKD. The American Journal of Kidney Diseases, 62(5), 849-859. doi:10.1053/j.ajkd.2013.06.008

[22] A. Makhlough, E. Ilali, R. Mohseni and S. Shahmohammadi. (2012). Effect of intradialytic aerobic exercise on serum electrolytes levels in hemodialysis patients. The Iranian Journal of Kidney Diseases, 6(2), 119-123.

[23] Centers for Disease Control and Prevention. Borg Rating of Perceived Exertion Scale. Retrieved from `https://www.cdc.gov/physicalactivity/basics/measuring/exertion.htm`. Accessed 17 September 2017.

[24] J. Wong, P. Davis, A. Patidar, Y. Zhang, E. Vilar, M. Finkelman and K. Farrington. (2017). The effect of intra-dialytic exercise on inflammation and blood endotoxin levels. Blood Purification, 44(1), 51-59. doi:10.1159/000455059

[25] K. Kalantar-Zadeh, J. D. Kopple, M. H. Humphreys and G. Block. (2004). Comparing outcome predictability of markers of malnutrition-inflammation complex syndrome in haemodialysis patients. Nephrology Dialysis Transplantation, 19(6), 1507-1519. doi:10.1093/ndt/gfh143

[26] E. Fiaccadori, A. Sabatino, F. Schito, F. Angella, M. Malagoli, M. Tucci, et al. (2014). Barriers to physical activity in chronic hemodialysis patients: a single-center pilot study in an Italian dialysis facility. Kidney and Blood Pressure Research, 39(2-3), 169-175. doi:10.1159/000355793

[27] G EuroQol. (1990). EuroQol-A new facility for the measurement of health-related quality of life. Health Policy, 16(3), 199-208.

[28] I. Al Salmi, A. Al Rukhaimi, A. AlSahow, F. A. M. Shaheen, S. M. G. Al-Ghamdi, F. Al-Ali, et al. (2016). Mineral bone mineral and its management among hemodialysis patients in the gulf cooperation council: Initial findings from the dialysis outcomes and practice patters study (2012-2015). Saudi Journal of Kidney Diseases and Transplantation 27(6 Suppl 1), S62-S80.

[29] F.S. Al-Ali, B. A. Bieber, R. L. Pisoni, H. Ezzat, M. AlGhonaim, F. AlHejaili, et al. (2016). Nutritional status and outcomes in hemodialysis patients from the gulf cooperation council countries enrolled in the dialysis outcome and practice patters study phase 5 (2012-2015). Saudi Journal of Kidney Diseases and Transplantation 27(6 Suppl 1), S31-S41.

[30] M. M. Bayoumi and, J. S. Al Wakeep. (2015). Impacts of exercise program on hemodialysis patients' quality of life and physical fitness. Quality in Primary Care, 23(4), 192-200.

[31] Dubai FAQs. Population of the UAE. Retrieved from www.dubaifaqs.com/population-of-uae.php (accessed August 24, 2017).

[32] M. Hecking, B. A. Bieber, J. Ethier, A. Kautzky-Willer, G. Sunder-Plassmann, M. D. Saemann, et al. (2014). Sex-specific differences in hemodialysis prevalence and practices and the male-to-female mortality rate: the Dialysis Outcomes and Practice Patterns Study (DOPPS). PLoS Med, 11(10), e1001750. doi:10.1371/journal.pmed.1001750

[33] Dubai Statistics Center. 2016. Percentage Distribution of Unemployed 15 years and over by nationality, sex and educational level - Emirate of Dubai. 2016. Retrieved from https://www.dsc.gov.ae/Report/DSC_LFS_2016_03_03.pdf (accessed September 25, 2017).

[34] M. Karavetian, S. Abboud, H. Elzein, S. Haydar and N. de Vries. (2014). Nutritional education for management of osteodystrophy (NEMO) trial: Design and patient characteristics, Lebanon. Nutrition Research and Practice, 8(1), 103-111. doi:10.4162/nrp.2014.8.1.103

[35] F. K. Port, R. L. Pisoni, J. Bommer, F. Locatelli, M. Jadoul, G. Eknoyan, et al. (2006). Improving outcomes for dialysis patients in the international Dialysis Outcomes and Practice Patterns Study. The Clinical Journal of the American Society of Nephrology, 1(2), 246-255. doi:10.2215/cjn.01050905

[36] P. A. Urena Torres. (2017). Strategies aiming to control hyperphosphatemia in chronic kidney disease. Néphrologie & Thérapeutique, 13 Suppl 1, S95-S101. doi:10.1016/j.nephro.2017.01.002

[37] A. White, H. X. Odedina, E. Campbell and R. Segal. (2006). The economic burden of end-stage renal disease with hyperphosphatemia. Disease Management & Health Outcomes, 14(2), 99-106.

[38] R. Rizk, M. Hiligsmann, M. Karavetian and S. M. Evers. (2016). Economic evaluations of interventions to manage hyperphosphataemia in adult haemodialysis patients: A systematic review. Nephrology (Carlton), 21(3), 178-187. doi:10.1111/nep.12584

[39] R. Rizk, M. Karavetian, M. Hiligsmann and S. Evers. (2017). Effect of stage-based education provided by dedicated dietitians on hyperphosphataemic haemodialysis patients: results from the Nutrition Education for Management of Osteodystrophy randomised controlled trial. Journal of Human Nutrition and Dietetics, 30(5), 554-562. doi:10.1111/jhn.12472

[40] A. A. Morais, M. A. Silva, J. Faintuch, E. J. Vidigal, R. A. Costa, D. C. Lyrio, et al (2005). Correlation of nutritional status and food intake in hemodialysis patients. Clinics (Sao Paulo), 60(3), 185-192. doi:/S1807-59322005000300002

[41] M. Karavetian, H. Elzein, R. Rizk, R. Jibai and N. de Vries. (2016). Nutritional education for management of osteodystrophy: Impact on serum phosphorus, quality of life, and malnutrition. Hemodialysis International, 20(3), 432-440. doi:10.1111/hdi.12405

[42] C. Moraes, S. M. Marinho, A. C. da Nobrega, B. de Oliveira Bessa, L. V. Jacobson, M. B. Stockler-Pinto, et al. (2014). Resistance exercise: A strategy to attenuate inflammation and protein-energy wasting in hemodialysis patients? International Urology and Nephrology, 46(8), 1655-1662. doi:10.1007/s11255-014-0712-3

[43] C. Delgado and K. L. Johansen. (2012). Barriers to exercise participation among dialysis patients. Nephrology Dialysis Transplantation, 27(3), 1152-1157. doi:10.1093/ndt/gfr404

[44] K. L. Johansen, G. K. Sakkas, J. Doyle, T. Shubert and R. A. Dudley (2003). Exercise counseling practices among nephrologists caring for patients on dialysis. The American Journal of Kidney Diseases, 41(1), 171-178. doi:10.1053/ajkd.2003.50001

[45] KDOQI. Clinical Practice Guideline for Hemodialysis Adequacy: 2015 update. (2015). The American Journal of Kidney Diseases, 66(5), 884-930. doi:10.1053/j.ajkd.2015.07.015

[46] S. H. Zyoud, D. N. Daraghmeh, D. O. Mezyed, R. L. Khdeir, M. N. Sawafta, N. A. Ayaseh, et al. (2016). Factors affecting quality of life in patients on haemodialysis: A cross-sectional study from Palestine. BMC Nephrology, 17(1), 44. doi:10.1186/s12882-016-0257-z

12

Effects of Caloric Restriction on Anthropometrical and Specific Performance in Highly trained University Judo Athletes

Lalia Chrara[1], Riad A. Raoui[1], Adel Belkadi[1], Hocine Asli[2], and Othman Benbernou[1]

[1]Laboratory for Optimising Research Programmes on Physical and Sports Activities, University of Mostaganem, Algeria
[2]Institute of Physical Education and Sport, University of Oran, Mostaganem, Algeria

Corresponding Author: Adel Belkadi; email: adel.belkadi@univ-mosta.dz

Abstract

Purpose: The purpose of this study was to determine the ultimate body mass, performance, and nutritional characteristics of the Algerian judo junior athletes, and also analysing the impact of nutritional intakes on stabilising Weight loss according to special performance of judo athletes. **Material:** 21 male university athletes (aged: 21.45 ± 1.32; height: 1.81 ± 0.45 m; and body mass: 73.9 ± 4.1 kg) participated in this study during a period of stabilising weight loss before and after 15 days of caloric restriction. Athletes were submitted to anthropometrical measurements and performed the Special Judo Fitness Test. Values for nutrient intakes were obtained from a 15-day food record kept during a training camp period of weight maintenance and after a 15-day caloric restriction. **Results:** Caloric restriction resulted in significant decreases in body mass (73.73 ± 2.1) and performance. However, Special Judo Fitness Test index increased significantly (14.00 ± 1.75) during caloric restriction in comparison to stabilising Weight loss. **Conclusion:** Exercise and caloric restriction lead to determine the ultimate weight and physical performance. The present study provides baseline nutritional data that can be used in the prescription of individual training programs for university judo Athletes.

Keywords: weight loss, nutritional, physical performance, judo

1. Introduction

Nutrition and Dietary is recommended as an important part of sport performance for young athletes [1]. Nutrition is increasingly recognized as a key component of optimal sporting performance, with both the science and practice of sports nutrition developing rapidly [2], Sports nutrition enhances athletic performance by decreasing fatigue and the risk of disease and injury; it also enables athletes to optimize training and recover faster [3], To optimize performance, young athletes need to learn what, when and how to eat and drink before, during and after activity [1]. [4] propose that high quality

Weight loss is often of importance to elite athletes in order to maintain their muscle (engine) and shed unwanted fat mass, potentially improving athletic performance

Judo is an intermittent combative sport requiring technical, tactical, and psychological skill that creates great muscle-strength and -power demands on both the upper and lower body [5]. Judo competitions are divided into weight classes. However, most athletes reduce their body weight in a few days before competition in order to obtain a competitive advantage over lighter opponents [6], and no study investigated a Weight loss higher than 5% of athlete's body mass. To achieve fast weight reduction, athletes use a number of aggressive nutritional strategies so many of them place themselves at a high health-injury risk [7]. Judo, as a combat sport, involves open and complex skills [8, 9], presenting irregular intervals of effort and pause, and characterized as an intermittent activity [5, 10, 11], However, few athletes maintain their daily body weight within the limits of their class before competition [12].

Weight loss is one of the most commonly used strategies by athletes in combat sports to gain a winning edge in their targeted weight classes [13]. The loss of large amounts of body mass in a short time is extremely harmful to the body; it can reduce muscle strength [14] also demonstrate that the exercise-induced hyperthermia and dehydration in the present experiments had only minor effects on the neuromuscular performance. In addition, reductions in renal blood fluid and the volume of liquid filtered by the kidneys [15, 16].Additionally, these physiological alterations can decrease anaerobic capacity, an important determinant of overall performance in judo [17]. A questionnaire was designed to evaluate rapid Weight loss patterns of competitive judo players and to assess its validity and reliability [18]. In conclusion, the questionnaire showed good validity and reliability and could be used accurately to assess Weight loss patterns of judo players. [19] concluded that weight reduction, consisting of both intense exercise and energy restriction, might possibly cause both an increase in oxidative burst activity and decrease in neutrophil phagocytic activity in judo athletes females. Additionally, studies investigating the effects of Weight loss on performance used at laboratory-based techniques [20], which may not reflect the demands of real judo combat heart rate [21, 22]. Therefore, a judo-specific performance test (Special Judo Fitness Test, SJFT), which is more representative of judo movements than laboratory tests, has been proposed as a valid and reliable measure of performance in judo athletes [8, 23–27].

2. Materials and Methods

2.1. Participants

Twenty-one healthy male university judo competitors took part in this study (mean (±SD); aged: 21.5 ± 0.7 years; height: 1.81 ± 0.45 m; and body mass: 75.0 ± 2.8 kg) participated in the study after receiving a comprehensive explanation of the procedure. This study protocol was in accordance with the Helsinki Declaration for human experimentation [28] and was approved by the scientific institute of sports ethics committee. The participants were also selected based on their mean period of practising judo was 9.2 ± 2.1 years. They competed in categories between -66 kg and -73 kg. Based on the results of a self-reported questionnaire, no subject had been treated with any experienced acute illness from infection during the first three months. Subjects reported no sleep disorder and did not consume any alcoholic beverages and none of them was taking any medication. All judokas participated in official judo competitions during this year and trained for 20-22 hours per week.

2.2. Study design

During the week before the experimentation, participants came to the training GYM several times to become fully familiarized with the procedure and tests involved so as to minimize learning effects during the experimentation. Athletes participated in two experimental test sessions. The first was a baseline condition in which athletes were taking a normal diet (baseline). The second was a condition of caloric restriction for 15 days; participants reduced their energy intake by 4.5 MJ/day (CR). At the end of each phase athletes performed the SJFT at the same time of day (10 a.m.). All experimental study were scheduled during a period with no official competitions.

At the end of each phase body mass, percent body fat, fat mass, fat-free mass, and body water were recorded using bioelectrical impedance scale to the nearest 0.1 kg (Tanita, Tokyo, Japan) calibrated in accordance with the manufacturer's guidelines by one trained technician. The body mass index was then calculated according to [29]. Following this, duplicate measurements were taken with participants standing and wearing only briefs, as recommended by the guidelines. The average of these two measurements was used for the final analysis. Moreover, the heart rate was monitored using Automatic Blood Pressure [30]. During the experimental period, participants were required to maintain their habitual physical activity and to avoid exhausting physical efforts 24 h before each test time.

2.3. Assessment of dietary intake

Nutritional assessment was carried out every 7 days to assess the energy intake of the subjects (i.e., fat, protein, and carbohydrate). Each athlete received recommendations needed to properly complete the food diaries. The athletes completed a self-administered validated Rapid Weight loss Questionnaire [13]. Thus, they detailed the food and beverages consumed during the 3 days prior to sampling. We asked athletes to maintain their normal diet during the study period (control period). Values for nutrient intakes were obtained from a food diary for a holding period of body mass and dietary restriction after 15 days. The plan was to carry out dietary restriction according to the report from [31]. The Weight loss methods used by athletes in this study appear to be generally used [32]. The records were analysed by a nutritionist using a computerized nutrition system, the NUTRISOFT- BILNUT [Vers. 2.01, Paris, France,33].

2.3.1. Special Judo Fitness Test (SJFT)

This test was proposed by Sterkowicz (1995). Briefly, three athletes of similar body mass are needed to perform the Special Judo Fitness Test: 1 participant (tori) is evaluated, and 2 other individuals receive throws (ukes). The tori begins the test in a position between the 2 ukes who are standing 6 m away from each other. On a signal, the tori runs to one of the ukes and employs a throwing technique called ippon-seoi-nage. The tori then immediately runs to the other uke and completes another throw. The athlete must complete as many throws as possible within the test time.

The Special Judo Fitness Test is composed of 3 periods (15 s, 30 s, and 30 s) separated by 10 s recovery intervals. Performance is determined by the total number of throws completed during each of the 3 periods. Heart rate is measured immediately after and 1 minute after the test and the following index is calculated as follows:

$$\text{SJFT Index} = \frac{\text{Final HR}(\text{b}\cdot\text{min}^{-1}) + \text{HR1min}(\text{b}\cdot\text{min}^{-1})}{\text{Throws(N)}}$$

where Final HR is the heart rate measured immediately after the test, HR 1 min is the heart rate measured 1 min after the test, and throws represent the total number of throws executed during the three sets.

2.4. Statistical analyses

The Levene test was used to check the homoscedasticity, and the Shapiro-Wilk test was used to test the normality of data, and given these assumptions were confirmed parametric statistics were used. Data are reported as mean ± SD, and 95% confidence intervals (95%CI) of the difference. Energy intake, anthropometric parameters, performance of SJFT, and heart rate were tested by a paired Student's *t*-test. The level of statistical significance was set at 5%. Cohen's d was calculated as post caloric restriction mean minus baseline mean divided by baseline standard deviation and classified according to Rhea (2004) for highly trained athletes (trivial < 0.25; small = 0.25 to 0.50; moderate = > 0.50 to 1.0; large = > 1.0).

3. Results

TABLE 1: Anthropometric parameters and daily nutrient consumption at baseline and caloric restriction periods (values are mean and standard deviation; n = 21).

	Baseline	Caloric restriction
Body mass (kg)	75.0 ± 2.8	73.73 ± 2.1*
Body water (kg)	42.7 ± 2.9	39.8 ± 3.6*
Body mass index (kg/m^2)	27.8 ± 2.4	26.8 ± 3.1*
Body fat (kg)	9.1 ± 2.2	8.8 ± 2.5
Free fat mass (kg)	66.8 ± 3.2	65.8 ±3.6*
Energy intake (kcal/day)	3675 ± 263	2274 ± 216*
Carbohydrates (g/day)	425 ± 39	264 ± 25*
Protein (g/day)	150 ± 11	87 ± 7*
Fat (g/day)	233 ± 10	92 ± 6*
Note: * Significant difference from baseline (p < 0.001).		

There was a significant effect of caloric restriction on body mass (t_{20} = 4.21, p < 0.001, 95%CI difference = 0.6 to 1.8, d = 0.43 [small]), body mass index (t_{20} = 4.25, p < 0.001, 95%CI difference = 0.51 to 1.50, d = 0.41 [small]), body water (t_{20} = 8.61, p < 0.001, 95%CI difference = 2.2 to 3.6, d = 1.00 [moderate]), fat free mass (t_{20} = 4.78, p < 0.001, 95%CI difference = 0.6 to 1.4, d = 0.31 [small]), energy intake (t_{20} = 16.35, p < 0.001, 95%CI difference = 1223 to 1580, d = 5.32 [large]), carbohydrate intake (t_{20}

= 14.67, $p < 0.001$, 95%CI difference = 138 to 184, d = 4.12 [large]), protein intake (t20 = 22.75, $p < 0.001$, 95%CI difference = 57 to 69, d = 5.70 [large]), and fat intake (t20 = 55.12, $p < 0.001$, 95%CI difference = 136 to 146, d = 14.00 [large]), with a decrease during caloric restriction compared to baseline. However, no change between periods was detected for body fat (t20 = 0.95, $p = 0.352$, 95%CI difference = −0.4 to 1.0, d = 0.13 [trivial]).

TABLE 2: Performance and heart rate responses during the Special Judo Fitness Test in judo athletes during normal diet (baseline) and after caloric restriction (values are mean and standard deviation; $n = 21$).

	Baseline	Caloric Restriction
A (rep)	5 ± 1	4 ± 1**
B (rep)	12 ± 2	12 ± 1
C (rep)	11 ± 2	10 ± 2
Total throws (rep)	28 ± 5	26 ± 3**
Final heart rate (bpm)	178 ± 6	189 ± 8**
Heart rate1min after (bpm)	163 ± 8	170 ± 8**
Special Judo Fitness Test index	12.72 ± 2.60	14.00 ± 1.75**

Note: A = first set of the Special Judo Fitness Test (15s); B and C = second and third, respectively, sets of the Special Judo Fitness Test (30s each); ** Significant different from baseline ($p < 0.01$); ** significant different from baseline ($p < 0.001$).

The caloric restriction resulted in significant decrease in the number of throws during A (t_{20} = 4.18, $p < 0.001$, 95%CI difference = 0.4 to 1.1, d = 0.80 [moderate]) and total (t_{20} = 3.05, $p = 0.001$, 95%CI difference = 0.5 to 2.9, d = 0.37 [small]) compared to the baseline, while increasing final heart rate (t_{20} = −6.71, $p < 0.001$, 95%CI difference = −14 to −8, d = −1.82 [large]), heart rate 1 min after the test (t_{20} = −8.26, $p < 0.001$, 95%CI difference = −9 to −5, d = −0.87 [moderate]) and index of the Special Judo Fitness Test (t_{20} = −3.77, $p = 0.001$, 95%CI difference = −2.00 to −0.58, d = −0.50 [moderate]) in the period of caloric restriction compared to baseline. No changes were observed concerning the number of throws in sets B and C.

4. Discussion

Our main aim in this study was to address the almost total lack of research evidence on stabilising Weight loss of judo athletes. We have done so by directly observing and reporting on the daily work of Twenty-one healthy male judo competitors, with special attention to their high judo training, caloric restriction whereby these assessments made themselves knowledgeable for all practical purposes, as dictated by their specific performance.

The main findings of the present study were that a 15-day caloric restriction program decreased judo athletes' body mass, body water, body mass index, free fat mass and judo-specific performance, specifically decreasing the number of throws during set A and total during the Special Judo Fitness Test, while increasing heart rate (after and 1-min after this test) and the index in this test (which indicates worse performance).The study [22] assess effectiveness of training's construction and of micro-cycle in total and detect in due time the trend to development of over-loading and failure of adaptation. As planned the caloric restriction program reduced total energy intake by 38%, resulting in decreased carbohydrate (38%), protein (42%) and fat (41%) intakes. However, this diet did not change body fat.

Despite the fact that athletes reduced only 1.7% of their body mass, which is in the range recommend for gradual Weight loss, performance was negatively affected. This is contrast to the observation that up to 5% rapid Weight loss did not affect judo-related performance [18]. Our findings are also different from those reported by [34] when comparing wrestlers and judo athletes submitted to gradual (5.0 ± 0.4% Weight loss in three weeks) or rapid Weight loss (6.0 ± 0.6% in 2.4 days). These authors reported no change in 30-m sprint and 1-min Wingate performances, suggesting that the athletes analysed coped well with both types of diets.

The ultimate goal is to identify a healthy body Weight that the athlete can maintain for most of the year, while minimizing the amount of Weight that needs to be lost for competition.

We hypothesized that the Weight loss would result in more detrimental effects on both caloric restriction and judo performance test. [16] investigate the effect of liquid losses occurring in training sessions during the competition period on some biochemical values of the male Judokas competing in the U18 category. The results of the performance tests support the fact that the duration of the intervention was important for changes in performance test. [35] Study results are equivocal when it comes to performance. Some studies report unchanged or improved performance in certain tests after Weight loss in athletes, despite loss of IBM [36]. There are several risks related to rapid Weight loss and Weight cycling, such as depressed immune activity [37–39], [40] indicate that supplying HMB promotes advantageous changes in body composition and stimulates an increase in aerobic and anaerobic capacity in combat sports athletes.

In this study, the caloric intake during the caloric restriction period leads to a significant decrease in body Weight (2.2 ± 0.23%), which was in accordance with other athletes in combat sports [41]. The loss of body Weight represented an average of 2.6

kg in absolute (Table 1).In this context, Artioli et al. [18] observed a reduction in body Weight after a 5-day Weight loss period when compared to control values. Likewise, Mendes et al. [42] showed a 5% reduction in body Weight after a 5-day Weight loss period. The most frequent methods used by judo players were increased exercise, restricted food ingestion, training in heated rooms, gradual dieting, and fluid restriction [43]. In accordance with several reports our results showed that rapid Weight loss affects negatively performance in judo athletes [44]. We herein argue that rapid Weight loss clearly meets all three criteria and, therefore, should be banned from the sport [45], Considering that these health-threating methods are more commonly used by lower level athletes, specific education programs should be directed to them [46]. In a recent review, Fagerberg [47] discussed the negative consequences of restricting calories too severely, [48] this review summarises guidelines for athletes and coaches for manipulating BM and optimising post weigh-in recovery, The ultimate goal is to identify a healthy body Weight that the athlete can maintain for most of the year, while minimizing the amount of Weight that needs to be lost for competition.

Although other studies analysed the effects of body Weight reduction on performance among combat sport athletes [12, 45, 46], it is worth noting that the present study was designed to determine the appropriate Weight. The Weight of an athlete can maintain without dieting is typically higher than their competition Weight [49]. The results of our study allowed us to conclude that stabilising Weight loss was not a good strategy to optimise judo athletes' performance. Finally, more research is needed concerning the long-term effects of stabilising Weight loss on physical and cognitive performance of judo athletes as recommended by [20], especially those investigating female judo athletes. also An individualized and well-planned gradual and safe Weight loss program under the supervision of a team of coaching staff, athletic trainers, sports nutritionists, and sports physicians is recommended. In addition, the sport dietitian can help make daily meal plans, address nutrition and sport supplements and health issues, and make sure the athletes is fuelled for their sport. This will improve their ability to design individualized and realistic Weight-management programs.

This study was limited by the reduced sample size of the population studied and the participants' characteristics as Olympic athletes, as well as the duration of the study (2weeks).

Another Two main limitations can be identified in our study: the absence of a control group submitted to a judo training and the lack of control concerning athletes' nutritional intake before the study. The use of control group in training camp is difficult, because athletes are submitted according to their performance result process. Additionally, some authors consider that there would be "ethical problems with restricting a particular treatment to elite athletes" [Atkinson, Nevill, 2001], athletes were not using any supplementation and were oriented to keep the nutritional training diet throughout the study.

Acknowledgments

The authors would like to thank the athletes who participated in the study for their time and patient. They would also like to thank the Algerian national coach and his staff and also Emerson Franchini for valuable contributions and careful proofreading. Thank you for your inspiration and for being a great friend and colleague.

Funding

Algerian Olympic Sports Centre and Institute of physical education and sports Sciences.

References

[1] Purcell, L. K. (2013). Sport nutrition for young athletes. Paediatrics & Child Health, vol. 18, no. 4, pp. 200–202. Available at: https://www.ncbi.nlm.nih.gov/pmc/articles/PMC3805623/

[2] Burke, L. M., Meyer, N. L., and, Pearce, J. (2013). National Nutritional Programs for the 2012 London Olympic Games: a systematic approach by three different countries. Nestlé Nutrition Institute Workshop Series, vol. 76, pp. 103–20.

[3] Hoch, A. Z., Goossen, K., and Kretschmer, T. (2008). Nutritional requirements of the child and teenage athlete. Physical Medicine and Rehabilitation Clinics of North America, vol. 19, no. 2, pp. 373–398, x.

[4] Hector, A. and Phillips, S. M. (2017). Protein recommendations for weight loss in elite athletes: A focus on body composition and performance. International Journal of Sport Nutrition and Exercise Metabolism, pp. 1–26.

[5] Ohya, T., Takashima, W., Hagiwara, M., et al. (2015). Physical fitness profile and differences between light, middle, and heavy weight-class groups of Japanese elite male wrestlers. International Journal of Wrestling Science, vol. 5, no. 1, pp. 42–46. Available at: https://doi.org/10.1080/21615667.2015.1030006

[6] Miarka, B., Branco, B. H. M., Vecchio, F. B. D., et al. (2015). Development and validation of a time-motion judo combat model based on the Markovian Processes. International Journal of Performance Analysis in Sport, vol. 15, no. 1, pp. 315–331. Available at: https://doi.org/10.1080/24748668.2015.11868795

[7] Artioli, G. G., Franchini, E., Nicastro, H., et al. (2010). The need of a weight management control program in judo: A proposal based on the successful case of wrestling. Journal of the International Society of Sports Nutrition, vol. 7, p. 15.

[8] Jagiello, W., Dornowski, M., and Wolska, B. (2014). Basic technical skills (throws) in 17-19-year-old judokas. Physical Education Studies, vol. 18, no. 6, pp. 77-80. Available at: https://sportedu.org.ua/index.php/PES/article/view/168

[9] Belkadi, A., Othman, B., Gleyse J, et al. (2015). Contribution to the identification of the professional skills profile of coaches in the Algerian sport judo system. International Journal of Sports Science, vol. 5, no. 4, pp. 145-150.

[10] Branco, B. H. M., Massuça, L. M., Andreato, L. V., et al. (2013). Association between the rating perceived exertion, heart rate and blood lactate in successive judo fights (randori). Asian Journal of Sports Medicine, vol. 4, no. 2, pp. 1251-30.

[11] Marcon, G., Franchini, E., Jardim, J. R., et al. (2010). Structural analysis of action and time in sports: Judo. Journal of Quantitative Analysis in Sports, vol. 6, no. 4, pp. 1–15. Available at: https://www.degruyter.com/dg/viewarticle.fullcontentlink:pdfeventlink/$002fj$002fjqas.2010.6.4$002fjqas.2010.6.4.1226$002fjqas.2010.6.4.1226.pdf?t:ac=j$002fjqas.2010.6.4$002fjqas.2010.6.4.1226$002fjqas.2010.6.4.1226.xml

[12] Abedelmalek, S., Chtourou, H., Souissi, N., et al. (2015). Caloric restriction effect on proinflammatory cytokines, growth hormone, and steroid hormone concentrations during exercise in judokas. Oxidative Medicine and Cellular Longevity, vol. 2015, p. 809492.

[13] NgQi, X., ChoeYee, X., Karppaya, H., et al. (2017). Rapid weight loss practices among elite combat sports athletes in Malaysia. Malaysian Journal of Nutrition, vol. 23, no. 2, pp. 199–209. Available at: https://www.cabdirect.org/cabdirect/abstract/20173365425

[14] Ftaiti, F., Grélot, L., Coudreuse, J. M., et al. (2001). Combined effect of heat stress, dehydration and exercise on neuromuscular function in humans. European Journal of Applied Physiology, vol. 84, no. 1–2, pp. 87–94. Available at: https://link.springer.com/article/10.1007/s004210000339

[15] Melin, B., Jimenez, C., Savourey, G., et al. (1997). Effects of hydration state on hormonal and renal responses during moderate exercise in the heat. European

Journal of Applied Physiology, vol. 76, no. 4, pp. 320–327.

[16] Çelik, N. M., Beyleroglu, M., Soyal, M., et al. (2017). The effect of liquid losses in trainings during competition period on some biochemical values of u18 male judokas (age 15–17). Physical Education of Students, vol. 21, no. 5, pp. 249–254. Available at: https://sportedu.org.ua/index.php/PES/article/view/488

[17] Filaire, E., Maso, F., Degoutte, F., et al. (2001). Food restriction, performance, psychological state and lipid values in judo athletes. International Journal of Sports Medicine, vol. 22, no. 06, pp. 454–459. Available at: http://www.thieme-connect.de/DOI/DOI?10.1055/s-2001-16244

[18] Artioli, G. G., Iglesias, R. T., Franchini, E., et al. (2010). Rapid weight loss followed by recovery time does not affect judo-related performance. Journal of Sports Sciences, vol. 28, no. 1, pp. 21–32. Available at: http://www.producao.usp.br/handle/BDPI/17423

[19] Suzuki, M., Nakaji, S., Umeda, T., et al. (2003). Effects of weight reduction on neutrophil phagocytic activity and oxidative burst activity in female judoists. Lumin Journal of Biological Chemistry Lumin, vol. 18, no. 4, pp. 214–217.

[20] Fortes, L. S., Costa, B. D. V., Paes, P. P., et al. (2017). Effect of rapid weight loss on physical performance in judo athletes: is rapid weight loss a help for judokas with weight problems? International Journal of Performance Analysis in Sport, vol. 17, no. 5, pp. 763–773. Available at: https://doi.org/10.1080/24748668.2017.1399323

[21] Villar, R., Gillis, J., Santana, G., et al. (2018). Association between anaerobic metabolic demands during simulated Brazilian Jiu-Jitsu combat and specific Jiu-Jitsu anaerobic performance test. The Journal of Strength and Conditioning Research, vol. 32, no. 2, p. 432. Available at: https://journals.lww.com/nsca-jscr/Abstract/2018/02000/Association_Between_Anaerobic_Metabolic_Demands.16.aspx

[22] Liu, Y. Q. (2015). Operative correction of judoists' training loads on the base of on-line monitoring of heart beats rate. Physical Education of Students, vol. 19, no. 2, pp. 13-21. Available at: https://sportedu.org.ua/index.php/PES/article/view/122

[23] Almansba, R., Franchini, E., and Sterkowicz, S. (2007). Uchi-komi avec charge, une approche physiologique d'un nouveau test spécifique au judo. Sci Sports, vol. 22, no. 5, pp. 216–223. Available at: http://www.sciencedirect.com/science/article/pii/S0765159707000731

[24] Artioli, G. G., Gualano, B., Coelho, D. F., et al. (2007). Does sodium-bicarbonate ingestion improve simulated judo performance? International Journal of Sport Nutrition and Exercise Metabolism, vol. 17, no. 2, pp. 206–217. Available at: http://journals.humankinetics.com/doi/abs/10.1123/ijsnem.17.2.206

[25] Degoutte, F., Jouanel, P., and Filaire, E. (2003). Energy demands during a judo match and recovery. British Journal of Sports Medicine, vol. 37, no. 3, pp. 245-249. Available at: https://www.ncbi.nlm.nih.gov/pmc/articles/PMC1724647/

[26] Detanico, D. and Santos, S. G. dos. (2012). Especific evaluation in judo: A review of methods. Brazilian Journal of Kinanthropometry and Human Performance, vol. 14, no. 6, pp. 738–748. Available at: https://periodicos.ufsc.br/index.php/rbcdh/article/view/1980-0037.2012v14n6p738

[27] Sterkowicz-Przybycien, K. L. and Fukuda, D. H. (2014). Establishing normative data for the special judo fitness test in female athletes using systematic review and meta-analysis. The Journal of Strength and Conditioning Research, vol. 28, no. 12, pp. 3585–3593. Available at: http://journals.lww.com/nsca-jscr/Abstract/2014/12000/Establishing_Normative_Data_for_the_Special_Judo.35.aspx

[28] World Medical Association. (2013). World Medical Association Declaration of Helsinki: ethical principles for medical research involving human subjects. JAMA, vol. 310, no. 20, pp. 2191–2194.

[29] Houcine, A., Ahmed, A., and Saddek, Z. (2014). Designing a software to count the body composition and somatotype and its role in pursing the morphological state of sportsmen. AASRI Procedia, vol. 8, pp. 38-43. Available at: http://www.sciencedirect.com/science/article/pii/S2212671614000742

[30] Elliott, K. E., McCall, K. L., Fike, D. S., et al. (2008). Assessment of manual blood pressure and heart rate measurement skills of pharmacy students: A follow-up investigation. American Journal of Pharmaceutical Education, vol. 72, no. 3. Available at: https://www.ncbi.nlm.nih.gov/pmc/articles/PMC2508710/

[31] Artioli, G. G., Scagliusi, F., Kashiwagura, D., et al. (2010). Development, validity and reliability of a questionnaire designed to evaluate rapid weight loss patterns in judo players. Scandinavian Journal of Medicine & Science in Sports, vol. 20, no. 1, e177–187.

[32] Shimizu, K., Aizawa, K., Suzuki, N., et al. (2011). Influences of weight loss on monocytes and T-Cell subpopulations in male judo athletes. The Journal of Strength and Conditioning Research, vol. 25, no. 7, p. 1943. Available at: https://journals.lww.com/nsca-jscr/Abstract/2011/07000/Influences_of_Weight_Loss_on_Monocytes_and_T_Cell.22.aspx

[33] Abedelmalek, S., Souissi, N., Takayuki, A., et al. (2011). Effect of acute maximal exercise on circulating levels of Interleukin-12 during Ramadan fasting. Asian Journal of Sports Medicine, vol. 2, no. 3, pp. 154–160. Available at: https://www.ncbi.nlm.nih.gov/pmc/articles/PMC3289209/

[34] Fogelholm, G. M., Koskinen, R., Laakso, J., et al. (1993). Gradual and rapid weight loss: Effects on nutrition and performance in male athletes. Medicine & Science in Sports & Exercise, vol. 25, no. 3, pp. 371–377.

[35] Garthe, I., Raastad, T., Refsnes, P. E., et al. (2011). Effect of two different weight-loss rates on body composition and strength and power-related performance in elite athletes. International Journal of Sport Nutrition and Exercise Metabolism. Available at: https://journals.humankinetics.com/doi/abs/10.1123/ijsnem.21.2.97

[36] Smith, M., Dyson, R., Hale, T., et al. (2001). The effects of restricted energy and fluid intake on simulated amateur boxing performance. International Journal of Sport Nutrition and Exercise Metabolism. Available at: https://journals.humankinetics.com/doi/abs/10.1123/ijsnem.11.2.238

[37] Imai, T., Seki, S., Dobashi, H., et al. (2002). Effect of weight loss on T-cell receptor-mediated T-cell function in elite athletes. Medicine & Science in Sports & Exercise, vol. 34, no. 2, pp. 245–250.

[38] Kowatari, K., Umeda, T., Shimoyama, T., et al. (2001). Exercise training and energy restriction decrease neutrophil phagocytic activity in judoists. Medicine & Science in Sports & Exercise, vol. 33, no. 4, pp. 519–524.

[39] Matthews, J. J. and Nicholas, C. (2017). Extreme rapid weight loss and rapid weight gain observed in UK mixed martial arts athletes preparing for competition. International Journal of Sport Nutrition and Exercise Metabolism. Available at: https://journals.humankinetics.com/doi/abs/10.1123/ijsnem.2016-0174

[40] Durkalec-Michalski, K., Jeszka, J., and Podgórski, T. (2017). The effect of a 12-week Beta-hydroxy-beta-methylbutyrate (HMB) supplementation on highly-trained combat sports athletes: A randomised, double-blind, placebo-controlled crossover study. Nutrients, vol. 9, no. 7, p. 753. Available at: http://www.mdpi.com/2072-6643/9/7/753

[41] Lopes-Silva, J. P., Felippe, L. J. C., Silva-Cavalcante, M. D., et al. (2014). Caffeine ingestion after rapid weight loss in judo athletes reduces perceived effort and increases plasma lactate concentration without improving performance. Nutrients, vol. 6, no. 7, pp. 2931–2945. Available at: http://www.mdpi.com/2072-6643/6/7/2931

[42] Mendes, S. H., Tritto, A. C., Guilherme, J. P. L. F., et al. (2013). Effect of rapid weight loss on performance in combat sport male athletes: Does adaptation to chronic weight cycling play a role? British Journal of Sports Medicine, bjsports-2013-092689. Available at: http://bjsm.bmj.com/content/early/2013/09/18/bjsports-2013-092689

[43] Artioli, G. G., Gualano, B., Franchini, E., et al. (2010). Prevalence, magnitude, and methods of rapid weight loss among judo competitors. Medicine & Science in Sports & Exercise, vol. 42, no. 3, pp. 436–442.

[44] Khodaee, M., Olewinski, L., Shadgan, B., et al. (2015). Rapid weight loss in sports with weight classes. Current Sports Medicine Reports, vol. 14, no. 6, p. 435. Available at: https://journals.lww.com/acsm-csmr/Abstract/2015/11000/Rapid_Weight_Loss_in_Sports_with_Weight_Classes.9.aspx

[45] Artioli, G. G., Saunders, B., Iglesias, R. T., et al. (2016). It is time to ban rapid weight loss from combat sports. Sports Medicine, vol. 46, no. 11, pp. 1579–1584. Available at: https://link.springer.com/article/10.1007/s40279-016-0541-x

[46] da Silva Santos, J. F., Takito, M. Y., Artioli, G. G., et al. (2016). Weight loss practices in Taekwondo athletes of different competitive levels. Journal of Exercise Rehabilitation, vol. 12, no. 3, pp. 202–208. Available at: https://www.ncbi.nlm.nih.gov/pmc/articles/PMC4934965/

[47] Fagerberg, P. (2017). Negative consequences of low energy availability in natural male bodybuilding: A review. International Journal of Sport Nutrition and Exercise Metabolism. Available at: https://journals.humankinetics.com/doi/abs/10.1123/ijsnem.2016-0332

[48] Reale, R., Slater, G., and Burke, L. M. (2017). Individualised dietary strategies for Olympic combat sports: Acute weight loss, recovery and competition nutrition. European Journal of Sport Science, vol. 17, no. 6, pp. 727–740.

[49] Manore, M. M. (2015). Weight management for athletes and active individuals: A Brief review. Sports medicine (Auckland, N.Z.), vol. 45, Suppl. 1, pp. 83–92. Available at: https://www.ncbi.nlm.nih.gov/pmc/articles/PMC4672016/

13

Food Safety Knowledge Among Chicken Shawerma Food Handlers in Amman-Jordan

Al-Nasraween M[1], Al Omari L[2], Al-Jaghbeer M[2], Al-Qutob R[2], Berggren V[3,4], and Taha H[2,3]

[1]Food and Drug Administration, Food Control Department, Amman, Jordan
[2]Community Health Department, Faculty of Medicine, University of Jordan, Amman, Jordan
[3]Faculty of Health Sciences, Lund University, Lund, Sweden
[4]Department of Neuroscience, caring science and society, Karolinska Institutet, Stockholm, Sweden

Corresponding Author: Taha H; email: hanagh@yahoo.com

Abstract

Aims. Several food poisoning outbreaks in Jordan were due to *Salmonella* species isolated from chicken shawerma. This study aimed to assess the food safety knowledge among chicken shawerma food handlers in Jordan. **Methods.** Forty chicken shawerma restaurants in Amman were selected randomly and 120 food handlers (Egyptians 53%, Jordanians 26% and Syrians 19%) were interviewed using a structured questionnaire. Descriptive and multivariate data analysis was conducted to assess their knowledge about food safety. **Results.** Low overall mean score of food safety knowledge (40%); the mean percent of correct answers about transportation, receiving of chicken shawerma, storage, preparation, selling, and controlling microorganisms were: 63%, 54%, 45%, 31%, and 26%, respectively. Ninety percent of the participants had no previous training in food safety concepts. Better food safety knowledge was significantly associated ($p > 0.05$) with higher educational levels, receiving special training in food safety and having a Jordanian nationality. **Conclusions.** This study recommends establishing a comprehensive food safety program in Jordan to build the capacity of the food handlers and enforce periodic evaluation of their food safety knowledge and evidence-based best practices.

Keywords: Food safety knowledge, Food handlers, Restaurants, Jordan

1. Introduction

The World Health Organization (WHO) emphasizes the importance of food safety as a global public health concern due to the rising number of food safety problems, coupled with recurring consumers' uncertainties [1]. Food-borne diseases can occur in any step of the long food chain cycle and people can get sick (Alhaddad et al., 2013; Azizieh, 2012; McIntyre et al., 2013; Osaili et al., 2013)]. Food handlers are considered one of the most important factors in the food chain since they come in direct contact with food during its transportation, storage, preparation and selling. Food-borne diseases can create an enormous burden on the economy, including medical, legal, and other expenses (Harakeh et al., 2005).

In Jordan most outbreaks of food poisoning have been attributed to *Salmonella* species isolated from chicken shawerma, which is consumed on a large scale by all classes of society (Kiswani and Nsour, 2007; Osaili et al., 2013). In 2007, the Jordan Food and Drug Administration (JFDA) set a new regulation of code of practices regarding handling shawerma (JFDA, 2007a). In the same year, a national food safety training program was initiated, and food handlers were compelled to get this training, especially those who work in shawerma restaurants. Unfortunately, this program was terminated with no justifiable reason. In 2010, the WHO published a comprehensive assessment of food safety in Jordan, that evaluation included major concerns about the health implications of poor knowledge and practices in food handling, limited human resources with food safety knowledge, inadequate consumer awareness and lack of regulation of street foods and food handlers [9]. Few studies were conducted in Jordan to estimate food handler's knowledge and practices. Osaili et al. published a study that aimed to assess the food safety knowledge among food workers in restaurants in Jordan (Osaili et al., 2013). The study revealed that the overall knowledge of food handlers on food safety concepts was fair. On the other hand, food handlers had poor knowledge about food-borne pathogens and safe storage, thawing, cooking and reheating of the foods but had good knowledge with regard to personal hygiene and symptoms of food-borne illnesses. Food handlers who received previous food safety training had a higher total food safety knowledge score than those who did not receive training.

Another study was conducted in Jordan by Sharif et al., which targeted 200 food handlers in military hospitals to assess their food hygiene knowledge, attitudes and practices [10]. The study found that food handlers in the military hospitals expressed high level of knowledge, positive attitudes and good practices in food safety. Still, there is a gap of knowledge in Jordan concerning the awareness of safety concepts among the workers in popular street food restaurants. Thus, this study aimed to investigate the food safety knowledge of chicken shawerma food handlers in Amman.

2. Methods

2.1. Settings

The Hashemite Kingdom of Jordan is divided into 12 governorates. Amman is considered the largest governorate in terms of its inhabitants, and it is the capital city of Jordan. Amman consists of 22 municipalities and has around 3070 restaurants. Out of these restaurants, there are 400 restaurants specialized in chicken and meat shawerma and they are distributed throughout the city as per the April, 2014 JFDA statistics (JFDA, 2014) .

2.2. Study design

A cross-sectional study was designed to conduct face-to-face interviews with chicken shawerma food handlers by using a structured questionnaire. The data collection took place in the period starting from 1 April 2014 until 30 June 2014.

2.3. Ethical approval

The ethical clearance for this study was issued by the University of Jordan Research Ethics Committee and the JFDA. Confidentiality and autonomy of the participants were insured. They were informed of the purpose of the study, the voluntary nature of their participation, and their right to access findings. Informed written consent was signed by all the participants. All the procedures performed in this study were in accordance with the ethical standards of the 1964 Helsinki declaration.

2.4. Food safety knowledge questionnaire

We developed the food safety knowledge questionnaire for this study based on the JFDA Shawerma food safety code of practice (JFDA, 2007b) and after an in-depth review of literature (Bolton et al., 2008; Municipality of Dubai, 2013; Osaili et al., 2013). The first part of the questionnaire was designed to collect socio-demographic characteristics, whereas the second section covered major food safety knowledge categories including safe food handling during:

- transportation and receiving of chicken shawerma (4 questions).
- storage of chicken shawerma (13 questions).
- preparation of chicken shawerma (18 questions).
- selling of chicken shawerma (12 questions).

In addition, there were 7 questions about the knowledge of controlling microorganisms' growth and multiplication in food.

2.5. Instrument validity and reliability

The food safety knowledge questionnaire was carefully examined by professors from renowned local universities. They checked the appropriateness of the questions and provided valuable comments. Furthermore 'Cronbach' alpha coefficient was used to find out the reliability of the food safety knowledge questionnaire.

2.6. Pilot study

The questionnaire was pilot tested by using a concurrent 'think -aloud' technique (Firestone, 1987) on 16 chicken shawerma food handlers for the purpose of seeking comments on the clarity of statements and length of time needed to complete the developed questionnaire. Questions were then modified to come up with the final version. The questionnaire was completed within 20 minutes by the food handlers.

2.7. Study sample

This study targeted the chicken shawerma food handlers in the 400 restaurants in Amman. Assuming that each restaurant has at least three food handlers involved in shawerma preparation; one is responsible for preparation of shawerma skewers and storage inside the operational room, the second is responsible for slicing the chicken shawerma while the third is responsible for preparing, wrapping, and selling sandwiches. Hence, the minimum number of shawerma food-handler workers in the 400 restaurants will come up to approximately 1,200 workers.

Geographical stratification was carried out for the 400 restaurants, then Percentage per geographical location of the restaurants was computed, the number of restaurants to be taken from each area was calculated using simple random sampling. A total of 40 restaurants were selected from each geographical area. After that, three food handlers were taken from each of these restaurants. The total sample of participants was 120 chicken shawerma food handlers.

2.8. Data collection

A total of 120 questionnaires were distributed among chicken shawerma food handlers to assess their food safety knowledge. The interviews were conducted by the first author to ensure that all the respondents equally understood the questions. All questionnaires were collected, making the response rate 100%. Upon checking and validating the collected questionnaires, 3 were discarded because of incomplete responses; hence the final sample was 117 participants.

2.9. Statistical analysis

The statistical analysis for this study was carried out using SPSS version 20. Descriptive data analysis was conducted (means, frequencies, and standard deviations). Student *t*-test, One-way Analysis of Variance (ANOVA), and Pearson correlation were used to assess the food safety knowledge and the associations between knowledge and various socio-demographic characteristics of the study participants. Fisher exact test was used for categories with < 5 frequency. P-value was set at < 0.05 to be considered statistically significant.

The knowledge level of chicken shawerma food handlers was calculated by adding the scores of correct answers in each category including transportation, receiving, storage, preparation, selling, and controlling microorganisms in chicken shawerma sandwiches. The Mean percent of total knowledge was calculated for each studied socio-demographic variable. Furthermore, standard deviation and significant association were computed. The total number of questions in all the categories was 54 questions. Each correct answer was given 1 score and incorrect answers or I do not know were given a 0 score. The highest possible score was 54. Independent sample *t*-test and One-way ANOVA test were used to compare the mean knowledge scores among different educational levels, nationality, and scope of experience of the food handlers.

3. Results

3.1. Study participants

Almost half of the participants were within 30–39 years age group. Of the participants in our study, 43% had diploma degree. More than half of the correspondents (53%) held the Egyptian nationality, while 26% were Jordanians, and 19% were Syrians. The majority of the food-handling workers (90%) did not receive training on food safety. Only 11% of the correspondents have been in the current job for 7 or more years, while 56% have been in the current job for 1–3 years. The socio-demographic characteristics of the respondents are presented in Table 1.

TABLE 1: Frequency and percentage of socio-demographic and personal characteristics of the respondents.

Characteristics		n	%
Educational level	Can read and write	3	2.6
	Elementary	3	2.6
	Preparatory	19	16
	Secondary	30	26
	Diploma	50	43
	Bachelor	12	10
Age	< 30	39	33
	30–39	57	49
	≥40	21	18
Nationality	Jordanian	30	26
	Egyptian	62	53
	Syrian	22	19
	Other	3	2.6
Experience in current job	1–3 years	65	56
	4–6 years	39	33
	≥ 7	13	11
Scope of past experience	In shawerma restaurants	44	38
	In restaurants in general	51	44
	Other	22	19
Years of past experience in food handling	≤ 5	69	59
	6–10	38	33
	≥ 11	10	8.5
Training in food safety	Has training	12	10
	No training	105	90

3.2. Food safety knowledge

This study tested the workers' knowledge in several elements concerning food safety in regards to transporting and receiving (Table 2), storing (Table 3), preparing (Table 4), selling (Table 5) and controlling microorganisms (Table 6) in chicken shawerma.

Regarding transportation and receiving of chicken shawerma, the percent average of correct responses was 63%. Although 97% of the correspondents believed that it is necessary to check the temperature of the transporting vehicle of chilled and frozen meat, only 45% and 39% knew the correct temperature of the transportation vehicle, respectively. Seventy-one percent of the correspondents knew the optimal time needed for transporting chicken shawerma prepared outside the restaurant from the chilled truck to the restaurant fridge.

The percent average of correct responses regarding optimal storage of chicken shawerma was 54%. Ninety-eight percent of the correspondents believed that it is necessary to check the temperature of the refrigerators and freezers in the restaurant. However, only 38% and 33% knew the correct running temperature of the refrigerators and freezers, respectively. Most of the correspondents (83%) believed that it is necessary to separate raw chicken from vegetables, but when they were asked about the correct place for storing vegetables in the refrigerator that is used also for storing/thawing meat, only 43% knew that vegetables should be stored in the upper shelves and meat should be stored in the lower shelves. The majority of the correspondents (98%) believed that it is necessary to cover marinated chicken in the refrigerators, however, only 50% knew that this practice is necessary to prevent cross contamination.

TABLE 2: Frequency and percent of the correct answers in food safety knowledge regarding storage of Chicken Shawerma.

Query Statement	*n*	**(%)**
1-Is it necessary to checkup the temperature of the fridge in your restaurant periodically?	115	98
2-What is the optimal temperature for storing chilled chicken?	44	38
3-What is the optimal temperature for storing frozen chicken?	39	33
4-In the chilling room with shelves for storing vegetables and chicken, where is the suitable place for storing chicken?	50	43
5-What is the dangerous temperature zone range in which the microorganisms multiply?	22	19
6-Is it necessary to cover the marinated chicken inside your fridge?	115	98
7-Why, it is necessary to cover the marinated chicken inside the fridge	59	50
8-If you have a food item in your restaurant with expiry date in the next month. What is the correct procedure from the following choices (i.e. Disposal 1st day of the month, last day of the month, return it to the supplier, or unsure)?	37	32
9-Is it safe to keep the shawerma skewer outside the fridge during summer without affecting its safety and quality?	41	35
10-Is it safe to keep the shawerma skewer outside the fridge during winter without affecting its safety and quality?	14	12
11-What are the signs of meat deterioration?	93	79
12-What is the best way to deal with the remnants of the shawerma skewer?	100	85
13- Is it necessary separate raw chicken from vegetables and other materials?	97	83
Mean % of correct answers to food safety knowledge in this category	54%	

Regarding the preparation of chicken shawerma, all the participants answered correctly that stainless steel or glass are best material of utensils for marinating chicken shawerma. However, only 54% of them correctly justified why they chose these materials. Only 7% of food handlers knew that frozen chicken was safer than fresh chicken.

Fifty-six percent of the correspondents knew that frozen meat should be thawed in the refrigerator but only 15% knew the optimal temperature of the shawarrma preparation room.

TABLE 3: Frequency and percent of the correct answers in food safety knowledge regarding Chicken Shawerma preparation.

Query Statement	*n*	%
1-What is safer to use for shawerma; frozen or chilled chicken?	8	6.8
2-If you choose either one in the previous question, why?	64	55
3-What is the safest method for thawing the frozen chicken?	66	56
4-If you thaw frozen chicken in the fridge, what is the optimal temperature for that?	20	17
5-What is the optimal temperature of the room where chicken shawerma is prepared?	17	15
6- What is the best source of water for preparing shawerma?	110	94
7-What is the best material of utensils for marinating chicken shawerma?	117	100
8-Why is stainless steel considered the best of these materials?	63	54
9-What is the maximum approved weight and diameter for the shawerma skewer by JFDA?	51	44
10-Is it important to distinguish knives used for chicken shawerma preparation from knives used for preparing other food items?	116	99
11-What is the best way for distinguishing knives used for chicken shawerma preparation from others?	14	12
12-Where is the best place for keeping shawerma skewer after preparation?	53	45
13-What is the optimal temperature for keeping chicken shawerma skewer?	17	15
14-What is the best way for cleaning utensils?	43	37
15- What is the best way for cleaning refrigerators?	44	38
16- What is the best way for cleaning hands?	43	37
17- What is the best way for cleaning tables before and after preparation of chicken shawerma?	37	32
18-What is the best and safest disinfectants of hands and tables?	71	61
Mean % of correct answers to food safety knowledge in this category	**45 %**	

The percent average of correct responses to questions about food safety in selling chicken shawerma was 30%. While 96% of food handlers answered correctly when asked about the necessity to wash their hands before using gloves, only 10% knew the best duration of hand washing as per the JFDA recommendations (for at least 20 seconds) .

The percent average of correct answers to the knowledge questions related to the effect of chilling and freezing on microorganisms was 26% (Table 5).

Total food safety knowledge scores were significantly (P <0.05) higher among respondents with bachelor's degree, had Jordanian nationality, and those who had previous training in food safety measures.

Table 4: Frequency and percent of the correct answers in food safety knowledge regarding selling of Chicken Shawerma.

Query Statement	*n*	%
1- Is it necessary to wash your hand before using gloves?	112	96
2- What is the best duration for hands washing?	12	10
3-Where is the best and safest place for knives sharpening?	28	24
4-What is the best way for knives cleaning after sharpening?	17	15
5-What is the best way for measuring the chicken shawerma temperature on the grill?	40	34
6-What is the safe temperature for chicken shawerma meat before serving?	24	21
7-What is the best way to know that chicken shawerma is well done and ready to serve?	14	12
8-If you are using forceps, is it necessary to wash your hands before serving.	115	98
9-What is in your opinion the best way for receiving the money from a customer?	11	9.4
10- Is it safe to use handmade mayonnaise? Why?	46	39
11- Where is the safest place for reserving sliced shawerma pieces?	4	3.4
12-What is the optimal temperature for keeping sliced chicken shawerma pieces?	9	7.6
Mean % of correct answers to food safety knowledge in this category	30%	

Table 5: Frequency and percent of the correct answers in food safety knowledge regarding controlling microorganisms in food.

Query Statement	*n*	%
1-Is there is a risk for microorganisms multiplication in shawerma?	113	97
2-What are the most common microorganisms responsible for food poisoning?	31	26
3- What are the bacteria types responsible for shawerma poisoning in Jordan?	40	34
4-What are the needed precautions to control microorganisms?	22	19
5-What is the effect of chilling on microorganisms?	2	1.7
6- What is the effect of freezing on microorganisms?	2	1.7
7-What is the time needed for microorganisms to multiply in optimal conditions?	5	4.2
Mean % of correct answers to food safety knowledge in this category	26%	

4. Discussion

The results of this study showed low overall food safety knowledge among the chicken shawerma handlers which is a matter of public health concern in Jordan. The participants had a relatively fair knowledge about food safety measures regarding transportation, receiving of chicken shawerma, storage and preparation. However, their knowledge scores were poorer regarding the safety measures during selling the

TABLE 6: Variations in the knowledge level of Chicken Shawerma food handlers across different educational levels, nationality, scope of experience and training in food safety.

Characteristics		*n*	Mean	% correct answers	SD	F	*p*-value
Education level	Bachelor	12	30.0833	56%	91.13991	3.154	0.011*
	Diploma	50	22.2000	41%	6.07437		
	Secondary	30	21.9474	41%	7.70281		
	preparatory	19	21.6667	40%	6.44182		
	elementary	3	20.6667	38%	2.51661		
	Write and read	3	20.000	37%	3.60555		
Nationality	Jordanian	30	27.3667	51%	9.40830	6.417	0.000*
	Egyptian	62	21.0645	39%	5.63325		
	Syrian	22	21.4545	40%	5.32494		
	Other	3	20.3333	38%	2.08167		
Scope of experience	In shawerma restaurants	44	23.0455	43%	7.35149	0.246	0.782
	Restaurants in general	51	22.8824	42%	7.87565		
	Other	22	21.7727	40%	5.00411		
Training	Has training	12	34.5000	64%	7.96013	5.543	0.000*
	No training	105	21.3905	40%	5.74204		

* *P*-value < 0.05, it is significant, meaning that the study have a significant association between variables.

n: Sample Size; SD = standard deviation = calculated value for ANOVA test; Significant value = *p*-value; Knowledge level % = (Mean /54).

chicken shawerma and controlling microorganisms. Higher overall food safety knowledge scores were found among respondents with bachelor's degree, had Jordanian nationality and those who had previous training in food safety measures.

In our study, only 10% of food handlers received training in food safety compared to a study conducted in Turkey, which revealed that 88.3% of food handlers received training on hygiene (Yard mc et al., 2015). Both studies show that those who have received training and are university graduates express the best knowledge on food handling safety measures (Yard mc et al., 2015). DeBess et al. also found that college graduates scored better on questions about safety measures (DeBess et al., 2009).

No significant relation was found between the years of experience food handlers had and their food safety knowledge, which is in concordance with the results obtained by Osaili et al. (Osaili et al., 2013).

Most of the food handlers (97%) knew it was necessary to check the temperature of chilled and frozen chicken trucks before receiving the chicken, but only 45% and 39% knew what the optimal temperature for chilled transportation and frozen transportation of food was. Moreover, it was found that 98% of food handlers believed that it was necessary to periodically check the temperature of the refrigerators at the restaurant, but only 38% and 33% of them knew what the optimal temperatures for storing chilled chicken and frozen chicken, respectively, were, similar to the results Onyrnrho and Hedberg (Onyeneho and Hedberg, 2013) obtained: only 38% of the participants knew the ideal refrigerator temperature. On the other hand, a study conducted in Ireland (Bolton et al., 2008) where 80% of food handlers received training in food safety showed that 97% of them knew the recommended temperature range for storing chilled and frozen food. This pattern of knowledge displayed by the food handlers we interviewed shows that most of them have a general idea about safety measures, but lack knowledge about the important specific guidelines because of the insufficient food safety training received.

We found that only 37% of food handlers knew the best way to clean their hands before preparing food, and 10% knew the best duration to wash their hands before selling food, which is significantly less than the result obtained by Osaili et al. (Osaili et al., 2013): 32% of their correspondents knew the best duration of hand-washing. The results obtained are alarming, as contaminated hands could contribute to the spreading of *Salmonella paratyphi A* (Nimri et al., 2014) and may be the main method of transmission of enteric viruses (Lillquist et al., 2005). However, a satisfactory 96% of correspondents knew that hands should be washed before wearing gloves.

Only 37% of food handlers knew the best way to clean utensils. This might be a major contributor to the spread of food-borne pathogens, as supported by the results of a study conducted in France by Gallay et al. (Gallay et al., 2008) that showed that poor utensil hygiene in the kitchen is a significant factor to acquiring *Campylobacter* infection.

Ninety-nine percent of the correspondents knew that it was important to distinguish knives used to prepare the chicken shawerma from other knives, but disconcertingly, only 12% of them knew how to do so. This could be a major contributor to cross-contamination, as revealed by Redmond et al. (Redmond et al., 2004).

The food handlers had the poorest knowledge regarding controlling microorganisms in food among other food safety measures (26%). Only 34% of the correspondents knew what the most common type of bacteria to cause food poisoning in Jordan is. Additionally, only 4.2% knew the time needed for microorganism to multiply in optimal conditions. These results emphasize the need for food safety training so that food handlers can know the different strains of pathogens found in different food types, the optimal conditions for microorganism growth, and the best methods to control microorganism and avoid contamination (Bolton et al., 2008).

In our study, overall food safety knowledge scores were higher among respondent with bachelor's degree, those that had a Jordanian nationality, and those who had previous training in food safety measures. The Social Cognitive Theory (SCT) states that behavior is shaped by the dynamic interaction between three determinants: behavioral, personal, and environmental influences (Versnik Nowak and Dorman, 2008). According to Bandura, self-efficacy construct of the SCT "refers to beliefs in one's capabilities to organize and execute the courses of action required to manage prospective situations" (Bandura, 1995). Educating and training food handlers about food safety measures and hygiene will undoubtedly increase their self-efficacy and contribute to better food management. Nieto-montenegro et al. found that the best approach to improve safety measures undertaken by food handlers is by combining standard training and social cognitive behavioral interventions (Nieto-montenegro et al., 2008). They suggest that to increase the effectiveness of a training program, food handlers' behavior, beliefs, and knowledge, and the interaction between these three factors must be understood, as well as by targeting the food handlers' motivational systems. Furthermore, they found that there was a beneficial outcome when supervisors adopted the position of role models.

Regarding personal influences, in a training program conducted by Soon and Baines, cases of victims of food poisoning were shared to improve the attitude of farm workers toward hand-washing by incorporating fear and enhancing risk perception (Soon and Baines, 2012).

As for environmental influences, Pilling et al. believe that adequate hand washing facilities and time will encourage food employees to wash their hands properly (Pilling et al., 2008). Moreover, food handlers should be reminded to perform food safety behavior (Pilling et al., 2008). Posters could serve as a proper reminder (Nieto-montenegro et al., 2008).

4.1. Strengths and limitations

The relatively small sample size of 120 food handlers is a limitation in this study. A larger sample size would have certainly contributed to more generalizable results, this was not feasible due to time and financial constraints.

This study was based on the assumption that there is a maximum of three food handlers involved in chicken shawerma preparation in every restaurant, which is not necessarily true. Ideally, all food handlers must be interviewed and their food knowledge assessed in order to get a better picture of the situation. However, this could not be performed because the restaurant owners did not allow all the employees to participate in the study as to not affect the restaurants' work flow.

The study covered the chicken shawerma restaurants in Amman only. Other provinces, which might probably have lower monitoring level of control by the supervisory authorities, where not addressed in the study.

The strength behind this cross-sectional study lies in the fact that it is a snapshot of a very specialized sector of restaurants that recorded the largest food-poisoning outbreak in the country, which has not been covered in any published article before. Moreover, to minimize the sampling bias, the restaurants were subjected to a geographical stratification, a percentage per geographical location was computed and a simple random sample amounting to 40 restaurants were selected from each geographical area, then three food handlers were taken from each of these restaurants.

There are some studies conducted in Jordan that have estimated food handler's knowledge and practices, but the uniqueness of this research resides in studying the preparation and selling of the shawerma sandwiches specifically. That is why the research team developed an exclusive questionnaire to assess the food safety knowledge of restaurant workers in this field.

The questionnaire covered all the processes of chicken-shawerma handling in order to provide a clear representation of the knowledge and practices of restaurant workers in this field.

5. Conclusion

This study revealed that food handlers' overall knowledge was poor in food safety issues that were assessed in the questionnaire. We assume that the poor knowledge of the workers will lead to incompliant practices, which could be a major contributing factor to a microbial contamination of the chicken shawerma sandwiches. Likewise, the statistical analysis of the collected data showed that there was a significant variation in the knowledge of chicken shawerma food handlers across different educational levels for the favor of bachelor degree holders. Our data also indicated that there was a significant variation seen in the assessment of the knowledge of chicken shawerma food handlers across different nationalities for the favor of the food handlers holding Jordanian nationality.

6. Recommendations

This study provided important data about the level of the knowledge of chicken shawerma food workers in Amman. We recommend further studies to investigate the impact of food safety knowledge among chicken shawerma food handlers' on their compliance with food safety practices. It is indisputable that poor knowledge about safety measures undertaken by food handlers is a major cause of food contamination and illnesses, and might yield future outbreaks of food poisoning. However, other factors play a role in food safety, including limited human resources, inadequate consumer awareness, the overlap of responsibilities across the food chain, the lack of multidisciplinary inspection teams and regulation of street foods and food handlers, and limited laboratory services (Nimri et al., 2014). All of these issues must be properly addressed to ensure food safety.

Therefore, this study proposes the following recommendations

The Ministry of Labor in Jordan must reconsider the instructions and regulations related to food handlers. For example, the workers must obtain training certificate in food safety before they start working in restaurants.

The food authority in Jordan must activate the training program which was provided for the shawerma food handlers and stated in the JFDA code of practice (JFDA, 2007b)(JFDA, 2007a). Furthermore, it should perform periodic evaluations for their knowledge and practices in a comprehensive food safety program by qualified trainers.

The media and newspapers must also participate in providing knowledge to the consumer on food safety.

Acknowledgements

The abstract of this study was accepted for poster presentation at the 11th European Public Health Conference, Ljubljana 2018. The authors thank the University of Jordan and the JFDA for supporting this research and the restaurants owners for granting them permission to interview the food handlers who voluntarily accepted to participate in this study. They would like to thank Prof. Kamel AL-Saleh for reading and commenting on the final draft of this manuscript.

Conflicts of Interest

All the authors declare that they have no conflicts of interest.

Availability of Data and Materials

The datasets generated and/or analyzed during the current study are not publicly available because of the confidentiality principle of the research project.

Funding

We thank the JFDA and the University of Jordan for funding this research.

References

[1] Alhaddad, A.S., Abushaala, F. A., and Bahout, A. A. (2013). Bacterial contamination of ready to eat foods (Shawerma Sandwiches) in Misurata City, Libya, in *2nd International Conference on Environment, Agriculture and Food Sciences (ICEAFS'2013)*, vol. 1, pp. 104–106. Available at: http://psrcentre.org/images/extraimages/513056.pdf

[2] Azizieh, A. (2012). Incidence and recovery of salmonella in chicken shawarma consumed in Damascus City and its countryside. *Damascus University Journal of Agricultural Science*, pp. 335–348.

[3] Bandura, A. (1995). *Self-efficacy in Changing Societies*. California: Cambridge University Press.

[4] Bolton, D. J., Meally, A., Blair, I. S., et al. (2008). Food safety knowledge of head chefs and catering managers in Ireland. *Food Control*, vol. 19, no. 3, pp. 291–300. DOI: http://dx.doi.org/10.1016/j.foodcont.2007.04.006

[5] DeBess, E. E., Pippert, E., Angulo, F. J., et al. (2009). Food handler assessment in Oregon. *Foodborne Pathogens and Disease*, vol. 6, no. 3, pp. 329–335. DOI: 10.1089/fpd.2008.0102

[6] FAO and WHO. (n.d.). *Pan-European Conference on Food Safety and Quality*. Available at: http://www.fao.org/docrep/meeting/004/x6865e.htm (accessed on April 28, 2018).

[7] Firestone, W. A. (1987). Meaning in method: The rhetoric of quantitative and qualitative research. *Educational Researcher*, vol. 16, no. 7, pp. 16–21. DOI: 10.3102/0013189x016007016

[8] Gallay, A., Bousquet, V., Siret, V., et al. (2008). Risk factors for acquiring sporadic Campylobacter infection in France: Results from a national case-control study. *The Journal of Infectious Diseases*, vol. 197, no. 10, pp. 1477–1484. DOI: 10.1086/587644

[9] Harakeh, S., Yassine, H., Gharios, M., et al. (2005). Isolation, molecular characterization and antimicrobial resistance patterns of Salmonella and Escherichia coli isolates from meat-based fast food in Lebanon. *Science of the Total Environment*, vol. 341, no. 1–3, pp. 33–44. DOI: 10.1016/j.scitotenv.2004.09.025

[10] JFDA. (2007a). Code of Practice in private shawarma restaurants for the year 2007.

[11] JFDA. (2007b). Code of Practice in private shawarma restaurants for the year 2007. Administration JF and D (ed.). Amman: JFDA.

[12] JFDA. (2014). Number of Restaurants in Amman.

[13] Kiswani, H. and Nsour, H. (2007). The curse of shawerma is chasing the government. *Al-Ghad Newspaper*.

[14] Lillquist, D., McCabe, M. and Church, K. (2005). A comparison of traditional handwashing training with active handwashing training in the food handler industry. *Journal of Environmental Health*, vol. 67, no. 6, pp. 13–16.

[15] McIntyre, L., Vallaster, L., Wilcott, L., et al. (2013) Evaluation of food safety knowledge, attitudes and self-reported hand washing practices in FOODSAFE trained and untrained food handlers in British Columbia, Canada. *Food Control*, vol. 30, no. 1, pp. 150–156. DOI: 10.1016/j.foodcont.2012.06.034

[16] Dubai Municipality. (2013). DG of Dubai Food Code. Available at: http://login.dm.gov.ae/wps/wcm/connect

[17] Nieto-montenegro, S., Brown, J. L., and Laborde, L. F. (2008). Development and assessment of pilot food safety educational materials and training strategies for Hispanic workers in the mushroom industry using the Health Action Model. *Food Control*, vol. 19, pp. 616–633. DOI: 10.1016/j.foodcont.2007.07.005

[18] Nimri, L., Al-Dahab, F. A., and Batchoun, R. (2014). Foodborne bacterial pathogens recovered from contaminated shawarma meat in northern Jordan. *Journal of Infection in Developing Countries*, vol. 8, no. 11, pp. 1407–1414. DOI: 10.3855/jidc.4368

[19] Onyeneho, S. N. and Hedberg, C. W. (2013). An assessment of food safety needs of restaurants in Owerri, Imo State, Nigeria. *International Journal of Environmental Research and Public Health*, vol. 10, no. 8, pp. 3296–3309. DOI: 10.3390/ijerph10083296

[20] Osaili, T. M., Abu Jamous, D. O., Obeidat, B. A., et al. (2013). Food safety knowledge among food workers in restaurants in Jordan. *Food Control*, vol. 31, no. 1, pp. 145–150. DOI: 10.1016/j.foodcont.2012.09.037

[21] Pilling, V. K., Brannon, L. A., Shanklin, C. W., et al. (2008). Identifying specific beliefs to target to improve restaurant employees' intentions for performing three important food safety behaviors. *Journal of the American Dietetic Association*, vol. 108, no. 6, pp. 991–997. DOI: 10.1016/j.jada.2008.03.014

[22] Redmond, E. C., Griffith, C. J., Slader, J., et al. (2004). Microbiological and observational analysis of cross contamination risks during domestic food preparation. *British Food Journal*, vol. 106, no. 8, pp. 581–597.

[23] Sharif, L., Obaidat, M. M., and Al-Dalalah, M.-R. (2013). Food hygiene knowledge, attitudes and practices of the food handlers in the military hospitals. *Food and Nutrition Sciences*, vol. 04, no. 03, pp. 245–251. DOI: 10.4236/fns.2013.43033

[24] Soon, J. M. and Baines, R. N. (2012). Food safety training and evaluation of handwashing intention among fresh produce farm workers. *Food Control*, vol. 23, no. 2, pp. 437–448. DOI: 10.1016/j.foodcont.2011.08.012

[25] Versnik Nowak, A. L. and Dorman, S. M. (2008). Social-cognitive predictors of college student use of complementary and alternative medicine. *American Journal of Health Education*, vol. 39, no. 2, pp. 80–90. DOI: 10.1080/19325037.2008.10599019

[26] WHO. (n.d.). Baseline information for food safety policy and measures – Estimating the Global Burden of Foodborne Diseases. Available at: http://www.who.int/foodsafety/about/flyer_foodborne_disease.pdf (accessed on April 28, 2018).

[27] Yard mc, H., Hakli, G., Cakiro lu, F. P., et al. (2015). Hygiene knowledge of food staff in catering industry: A sample From Turkey. *SAGE Open*, vol. 5, no. 2. DOI: 10.1177/2158244015580376

14

Physical Activities of Young Girls in Jeddah, Saudi Arabia

Elham A. Aljaaly

King Abdul-Aziz University, Saudi Arabia

Corresponding Author: Elham A. Aljaaly; email: ealjaaly@kau.edu.sa

Abstract

Background: Physical education classes are non-existent in Saudi girls' curriculum at all educational levels and physical activities are not permitted at public schools. The study aimed to assess physical activities for female students in intermediate and high schools.

Methods: A questionnaire was completed by 1519 participants from 18 schools in Jeddah City. Activities at school and after school were reported. About 63% of the girls preferred to have physical education classes at school.

Results: Girls thought that they were performing (43.2%) enough physical activities and (74%) rated themselves as performing an average level of physical activity in comparison with their peers. Only 32% linked the importance of physical activities to their health. Cars are the main transportation methods to and from school (87 %) and 8% walked to school. Some physical activities (59.2%) are performed at school [walking during break times (42%) or running (5.2%)]. Only 40% were involved in light activities after school while 54% participated in washing up or cleaning the house. Other activities outside school, e.g. walking, shopping, bowling, horse riding and table tennis was reported by 48% of the participants. Moderate activities such as swimming, cycling, dancing, or competitive running was reported by 70% of the respondents. Only 13% joining fitness centres.

Conclusion: Results emphasized the central role and obligation of decision makers in protecting young consumers through providing a healthy environment in schools.

Keywords: Physical activity, Schoolgirls, Weight status, Waist circumference, Saudi Arabia

1. Background

Previous research concerning the health of school children and youth aged 5–17 years conventionally concentrated on physical activity and exercise, with the evidence supporting the importance of meeting physical activity guidelines of 60 min of MVPA (moderate-to-vigorous physical activity) per day (Carson et al., 2016). Sedentary behaviour, where energy expenditure is ≤1.5 METs (metabolic equivalent), is currently a behaviour of particular importance [18]. Studies and reviews including Saudi [2] have abridged the benefits of regular physical activity on several health and behavioural outcomes of adolescents, and its potential for reducing the incidence of chronic diseases that are manifested in adulthood. In addition, risk factors associated with cardiovascular diseases in adolescence that includes overweight status, hypertension, increased blood lipids, and cholesterol are linked to physical inactivity [9]. Saudi children and adolescents (71%) do not meet the minimal weekly requirement of moderate to vigorous physical activity necessary for an effectively functioning cardiorespiratory system [3]. In Saudi Arabia television viewing, videos, and computer games were the factors which contributed most to the inactivity epidemic. Females are less involved in sports, exercise, and physical activity than boys [3, 11]. In Saudi Arabia, physical activities are not permitted at public schools for girls at all educational levels [5]. Physical education classes are also not fully considered in Saudi curriculum for girls [14], as these activities are still considered contrary to cultural and social norms and beliefs. Saudi girls infrequently use walking as a method of transportation to and from school, and many leisure activities, which are sedentary, including television (TV) and computer are used by teen girls after school (Aljaaly, 2012). Saudi girls have access to health and nutrition information through media, mainly TV (Taha, 2008). Despite the absence of sporting activities at schools for Saudi girls, health fitness centres are designed especially for females are available in most Saudi cities, and swimming pools exist inside some homes, particularly for wealthy families. Outdoor activities, such as, walking is prevalent, and many suitable and private places for out-of-doors activities were developed by the government in the last decade to encourage this behaviour. Jeddah is a waterfront city with a long (40 kilometres) coastline, which provides a perfect setting for outdoor activities (water and non-water oriented activities), although the hot and humid climate of Jeddah during most time of the year encourages individuals to participate in indoor rather than open-air activities. In the Saudi society it is still slightly banned for women to engage in many sporting and recreation activities [1]. In Saudi Arabia, women are required to wear "Abaya", which is the dress code for Saudi women and could limit outdoor activities or available options with respect to sport and recreation. This study aimed to assess physical activities for Saudi female students in intermediate and high schools. Associations with outcome measures such as weight status and waist circumference (WC) of participants with the concern and the practice of physical activities was also assessed and objectives were developed to identify associations between physical activities and nutritional status (based on weight categories and WC).

2. Methods

The study is part of a large cross-sectional survey that was conducted in 1519, participants aged 13 to 18-years-old. Eighteen schools were included in the study, aimed to assess the nutritional status of adolescents' girls. Detailed methods were previously published [7]. The present paper aimed to assess physical activities for female students in intermediate and high schools and explained with two objectives: to identify associations of participants' physical activities with weight categories (using the WHO 1995 guidelines for BMI classification by age and gender, which was stratified into two risk-based BMI categories (underweight and overweight) and WC at ≥ 75th percentile, according to Fernandez et al. in 2004 [6]. A questionnaire concerning perceptions and performance of physical activities was completed by participants and measures were derived from the self-completed questionnaires. Surveys were based on participants' observation and evaluation of their own activity levels. Activities included those done at different times in the day either at school, after school, at home, or in girls' free times (Var. 1-15) in Table 1. Information was collected using the guidelines of GPAQ [17], with modifications. Data on physical activities were designed, grouped and collected based on physical activity participation in three settings (or domains) as well as sedentary behaviours. The domains were activities at school (travels to and from school and apart from school), recreational activity which included activity performed after school, at home, or away from home (indoor or outdoor). Other survey data included sleep habits, a different types of physical activities and whether the student was involved in exercises, outdoor exercises or those at fitness centres or in their leisure times. Some of the activities were evaluated according to daily performances while others on weekly basis. Physical activity was divided into three levels: 1) Sedentary behaviours (sittings or reclining after school or at home). 2) Very light (activities those which require a lowest energy expenditure such as sleeping hours. 3) Very low energy activities such as television watching or playing on computer. 4) Light, moderate or hard activities (activities on a range of prompted activities that were known to require light, moderate, high or very high levels of energy expenditure). The grouping and classification of activity levels used was based on the 1997 UK Survey for young people with modification [15]. But, activities in this survey could be reported by girls as 'were occasionally performed' and not as 'being done regularly'. The Research Ethics Committee of at King Abdul-Aziz University reviewed the study protocol and granted approval. Permission to administer this survey at schools for girls was granted by School Health Department at Ministry of Education in Saudi Arabia. Information letters and consent forms were provided to students and their parents beforehand collecting data. This was in order to define the number of students with parental consents. Students who returned their letters completed and signed included in the survey. Mean, SD and percentages and chi square (at a significant levels of $p < 0.05$) were the statistical analyses used.

3. Results

The study confirmed that cars are the main transportation methods to and from school as (87 %) and 8% walked to school. Adolescent girls reported performing some physical activities (59.2%) at school. Schools' activities were reported as of walking during break times (42%) or running (5.2%) and the rest of students (12%) reported performance of both activities. Sedentary activities such as sitting down, eating and talking to their friends during school breaks were reported by 41%. Only 40% of girls were involved in light activities after school, e.g. food preparations while 54% participated in washing up or cleaning the house. Other activities outside school, e.g. walking, shopping, bowling, horse riding and table tennis was reported by 48% of the participants. Moderate activities such as swimming, cycling, dancing, or competitive running as jogging was reported by 70% of the respondents and 80% of these activities were more likely to be performed two times or more per week. Thirteen-percent of the participants afforded to join fitness centres to perform exercises and physical activities 'as it was not affordable for most of the girls for the high cost', which was mostly performed once a week. Participants reported concerns related to physical activities. For example, a high proportion (74%) of Jeddah girls thought that they were more active in comparison to peers and friends. About 63% of Saudi adolescent girls preferred to have physical education classes at school. Commonly, they reflected the same levels of physical activities in holidays, in comparison to school days, and (43.2%) of the participants considered they perform enough exercise to keep them healthy. Only 32% linked the importance of physical activities to their health.

Looking at the weight categories for the same population [7] (Figure 1), and when associating data with participants' performance and perceptions about physical activities, we found some differences in girls' weight status according to girls' perceptions of physical activity patterns, however no significant associations was found. This concerned all other association between weight status and different types of physical activities. The overweight girls were also more likely to consider their levels of physical activity as an average in comparison to others in the same age, compared to underweight girls. Sedentary behaviours (reading and use of other media sources) were not associated with any particular weight status.

The survey findings suggested that waist circumference measurements were also significantly associated with girls' physical activity **(Table 2).** Girls with large WC

NO	VARIABLE NAME	LABEL	INDICATORS
1	**PA_ Holidays**	During holidays, how active are you in comparison to school days?	Three categories: Less active, about the same, more active
2	**Enough_ Exercises**	In general speaking, do you think that you perform enough exercise to keep healthy?	Two categories: Yes, NO
3	**Enough excercise_holidays**	Do you perform enough physical activities during holidays in comparison to school days?	Three categories: less active, about the same, more active,
4	**Active._ compare**	How active are you, in comparison to others your age and sex?	Three categories: Below average, about average, above average
5	**Ph_ education_ classes**	Would you prefer to have physical education classes at school?	Two categories: Yes, NO
6	**Go _bed_ Early**	Do you normally go to bed early?	Two categories: Yes, NO
7	**Getup_ Early**	Do you normally get up early?	Two categories: Yes, NO
8	**Transportations_ Type**	Which type of transportation do you use for school and apart from school?	Three categories: car, walk, public transport
9	**PA_ at_ School**	Do you usually do any kind of PA at school?	Two categories: Yes, NO
10	**PA_ School_ Breaks**	What do you usually do at school breaks?	Three categories: sitting down, standing or walking around, running or other PA
11	**Reading_ Hours**	How many hours/day do spend in reading books, magazines, or comics?	Two categories: less than 2 hour/day, Or 2 hrs or more/day
12	**Homework_ Time**	How many hours per day do you spend on doing your homework?	Two categories: less than 2 hour/day, Or 2 hrs or more/day
13	**TV_ Hours**	How many hours/day do you spend watching TV or video?	Two categories: less than 2 hour/day, Or 2 hrs or more/day
14	**Playing_ Computer/ Computer_ Games**	How many hours/day do you spend on Computer or computer games?	Two categories: less than 2 hour/day, Or 2 hrs or more/day
15	**Light_ PA _Outside_ School**	Do you normally perform any kind of physical activities outside school e.g. walking, shopping, bowling, horse riding, and table tennis?	Two categories: Yes, NO

TABLE 1: Variables and Measures for Physical Activities. Perceptions, knowledge, attitudes variables about physical activities

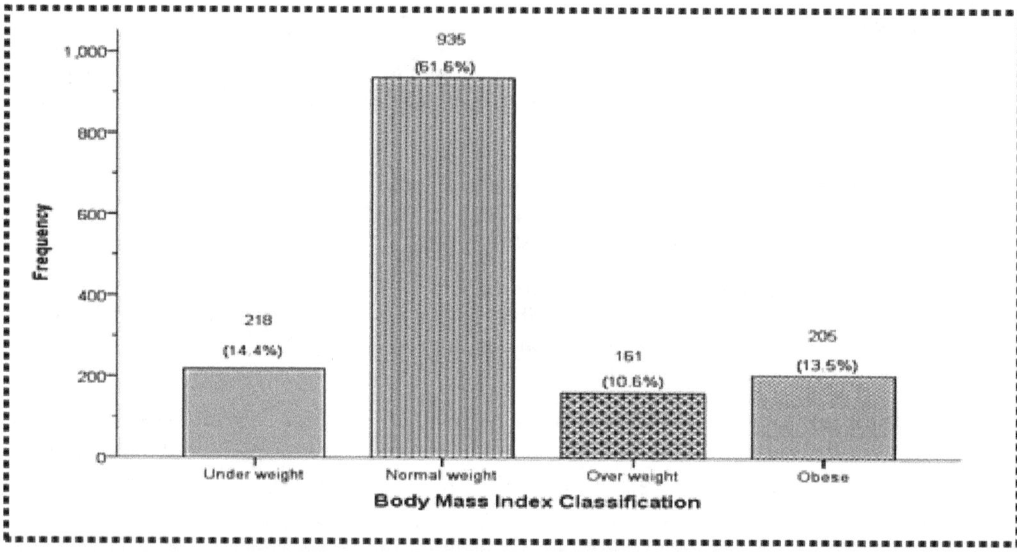

Figure 1: Weight status for participants. Source [7].

thought that they were more active outside school compared to inside school, and they were performing more activities outside school. They also most likely considered themselves healthy and reported performance of moderate activities, compared to those who had lower waist size (<75th percentile).

4. Discussion

Participants reported concerns related to physical activities and a high proportion of Jeddah girls thought that they were more active in comparison to peers and friends. Commonly, they reflected the same levels of physical activities in holidays, in comparison to school days, and most of the participants considered themselves performing enough exercise to keep them healthy. Findings confirmed no significant associations for physical activities with weight status based on other indices such as BMI status. This is in agreement with Fayssal et al., [1], who found that physical activity at different levels did not significantly relate to BMI on the 12-19 years-old population from three different provinces, including the Western province of Saudi Arabia. Girls with greater waist size were more likely to perform physical activities outside the school environment, and to perform moderate activities such as cycling and swimming, compared to those with lower WC at the 75th percentile.

Variables (number of respondents)	[WC at 75th percentile cut-off point]		
* Data reflects positive response	WC <75th n (%)	WC ≥75th n (%)	P Values
During holidays, how active are you in comparison to school days? (1511)			*P* = 0.005
Less active (534)	220 (38.3)	314 (33.5)	
About the same (325)	137 (23.8)	188 (20.1)	
More active (652)	218 (37.9)	434 (46.4)	
Do you normally perform any kind of physical activity outside school? (1484)*	369 (35.1)	673 (73.6)	*P*<0.001
Do you perform physical activities like: cycling, tennis, bowling, and horse-riding? (1476)*	141 (25)	294 (32.2)	*P*= . 003
In general speaking, do you think that you perform enough exercise to keep healthy (1504)*	161 (28.1)	388 (33.9)	*P* = .006

TABLE 2: Comparisons between surveys about physical activities & WC. WC at 75th percentile cut-off point.

5. Conclusion & Recommendations

1. Results emphasized the central role and obligation of decision makers in protecting young girls through providing a healthy environment in schools, which will affect girls' activities even after school.

2. Educational classes including physical education should be included in adolescent girls' schools, to enhance their knowledge and perceptions about the importance of physical activities in their life.

3. In order to achieve goals of this study, policy makers need to include physical education and activities in public schools to enhance girls' performance for physical activities and to acquire health benefits out of this activities.

6. Conflict of Interests

The author declares that there is no conflict of interests regarding the publication/presentation of this work.

References

[1] M. Abou El-Ela, M. Soliman, and M. Amin, "Urban Waterfronts between Cultural and Physical Influences (The case of Jeddah and Alexandria) ," in *international sociaty of city and regional planning Conference - 43rd Isocarp Congress*, Belgium, 2007.

[2] S. Al-Ghamdi, "The association between watching television and obesity in children of school-age in Saudi Arabia," *Journal of Family and Community Medicine (JFCM)*, vol. 20, no. 2, p. 83, 2013.

[3] H. M. Al-Hazzaa, "Physical activity, fitness and fatness among Saudi children and adolescents: Implications for cardiovascular health," *Saudi Medical Journal*, vol. 23, no. 2, pp. 144–150, 2002.

[4] H. M. Al-Hazzaa, N. A. Abahussain, H. I. Al-Sobayel, D. M. Qahwaji, and A. O. Musaiger, "Lifestyle factors associated with overweight and obesity among Saudi adolescents," *BMC Public Health*, vol. 12, no. 1, article 354, 2012.

[5] E. Aljaaly, "Personal and Environmental Influences on Eating Behaviours of Adolescent Girls in Saudi Arabia," in *World Sustainable Development Outlook 2015 Green Behavior: Re-thinking Policy for Sustainability*, 2015, ISBN: 978-1-907106-35-4; ISSN 1748-8133.

[6] E. Aljaaly, "Centralized fat status of adolescent girls in Saudi Arabia in comparison to the United Kingdom Reference Data," *British Journal of Medical and Health Research*, vol. 1, no. 3, 2014.

[7] E. Al-Jaaly, M. Lawson, and T. Hesketh, "Overweight and its determinants in adolescent girls in Jeddah City, Saudi Arabia," *IJFNPH*, vol. 4, no. 2, pp. 95–108, 2011.

[8] E. Al-Jaaly, *Factors affecting nutritional status and eating behaviours of adolescent girls in Saudi Arabia [Ph.D. thesis]*, London, UK, UCL, 2012, http://discovery.ucl.

[9] B. A. Spear, "Adolescent growth and development.," *Journal of the Academy of Nutrition and Dietetics*, vol. 102, no. 3, pp. S23–S29, 2002.

[10] V. Carson, S. Hunter, N. Kuzik et al., "Systematic review of sedentary behaviour and health indicators in school-aged children and youth: An update," *Applied Physiology, Nutrition, and Metabolism*, vol. 41, no. 6, pp. S240–S265, 2016.

[11] F. M. Farahat, K. P. Joshi, and F. F. Al-Mazrou, "Assessment of nutritional status and lifestyle pattern among Saudi Arabian school children," *Saudi Medical Journal*, vol. 28, no. 8, pp. 1298–1300, 2007.

[12] J. R. Fernández, D. T. Redden, A. Pietrobelli, and D. B. Allison, "Waist circumference percentiles in nationally representative samples of African-American, European-American, and Mexican-American children and adolescents," *Journal of Pediatrics*, vol. 145, no. 4, pp. 439–444, 2004.

[13] D. Taha, O. Ahmed, and B. B. Sadiq, "The prevalence of metabolic syndrome and cardiovascular risk factors in a group of obese Saudi children and adolescents: A hospital-based study," *Annals of Saudi Medicine*, vol. 29, no. 5, pp. 357–360, 2009.

[14] A. Musaiger, N. Zagzouk, and M. Almaaie, "The nutrition habits. Life style and obesity among adolescents in Jeddah city. Saudi Arabia (A comparison between governmental and private schools). ," in *The second conference of obesity*, Bahrain, 2005, [Published paper in conference booklet].

[15] G. Smithers, C. J. Gregory Bates Jr, A. Prentice, L. V. Jackson, and R. Wenlock, "The National Diet and Nutrition," *The National Diet and Nutrition*, 2000.

[16] D. Sellen, "Physical Status: The Use and Interpretation of Anthropometry. Report of a WHO Expert Committee. WHO Technical Report Series No. 854. Pp. 452. (WHO, Geneva, 1995.) Swiss Fr 71.00.," *Journal of Biosocial Science*, vol. 30, no. 1, pp. 135–144.

[17] T. Armstrong and F. Bull, "Development of the World Health Organization Global Physical Activity Questionnaire (GPAQ)," *Journal of Public Health*, vol. 14, no. 2, pp. 66–70, 2006.

[18] T. Yates, E. G. Wilmot, and M. J. Davies, "Sedentary behaviour: Whats in a definition?" *Am J Prev Med*, vol. 40, pp. e33–10, 2011.

15

Effects of Dietary Fiber Intake on Body Weight and Waist Circumference

Eiman Al Hammadi

Department of Natural Sciences and Public Health, Zayed University, Abudhabi, UAE

Corresponding Author: Eiman Al Hammadi; email: eimanal-hammadi@hotmail.com

Abstract

Aim: Obesity levels dramatically increased in the last decade in UAE. Diets high in energy, saturated fatty acids, low intake of fruits and vegetables as well as inactivity have been found to promote overweight and obesity. A diet high in fiber has been suggested to improve weight loss and decrease other anthropometrical indices. The purpose of this study was to assess the effect of a diet high in fiber on body weight, BMI, and waist circumference (WC).

Methods: One hundred forty overweight/obese subjects aged from 20-30 years old participated in the study. Body weight (BW), body mass index (BMI) and waist circumference (WC) was measured after one month period in which the subjects consumed diet high in dietary fiber (38 g/d/men, 25 g/d/women). SPSS was used for the analysis of data and statistically significant difference was set at $P > 0.05$.

Results: BW, BMI and WC were clinically reduced before and after intervention in both males and females. However, these changes were not statistically significant. Percent changes on BW for female and male subjects were 1.45 (95%CI: -12.68, 15.58), $P > 0.05$ and 1.12 (95% CI: -13.58, 15.82), $P > 0.05$, respectively.

Conclusion: The high fiber diet did not significantly reduce body weight and WC. Even though there was a small clinically reduction on BW, BMI and WC, however this was not statistically significant. The results, even though were not supportive, they should not discourage people from consuming foods high in fiber, due to other beneficial effects in their health such as decreasing the risk of cancer, lipidemia, type 2 diabetes and metabolic syndrome.

Keywords: Dietary fiber; weight loss; body mass index; waist circumference

1. Introduction

The problem of overweight and obesity have gone to high proportions globally, besides one of the reasons is adoption of a westernized lifestyle, intake of excessive food and inadequate physical activity are common characteristics of this life style [1]. References in the last two decades indicate that obesity has reached to double in USA, and now 30% of the US adult population is classified as obese, while the overweight people are reaching the 35%. Pediatric obesity is also an increasing problem with about 16% being overweight and an additional 15% are at risk of overweight [2].

In addition, increased levels of obesity and low physical activity has been noted during these decades, with shocking increases in prevalence of type 2 diabetes. The number of the total adults with diabetes type 2 is expected to be doubled between 2000 and 2030 [2].

The prevalence of obesity is high in industrialized societies. According to research report by CDC [3] "more than one-third of U.S. adults (34.9%) are obese while the annual medical cost of obesity in the U.S. is $147 billion" [3].

A report published by the Gulf News (July, 2012) referring to BMC Public Health journal published in the health journal warned that the world's adult population is getting fatter rapidly. 17 million tones of total population weight are due to people being overweight [4].

UAE Ministry of Health had warned that more people are dying of non-communicable diseases such high blood pressure, diabetic and heart failure. The ministry alarmed that children are less physically active today which will make population obese by the year 2015. According to the ministry sources about 44.5 % of the women in the UAE could become obese in coming years if it goes on the same rate as today [5].

In UAE obesity is not only a problem in women and men but this is increasing in children also. One of the common reasons of obesity in children UAE is changing eating habits revealed in their research that the influx of the Western lifestyle [6]. This life style has resulted in changes in both behavioral patterns and food consumption habits. The traditional style of eating and foods such as milk, dates and porridge is being replaced by processed foods such as soda, high sugar, and high fat foods items [7].

Dietary fiber can be metabolized by the gut micro biota to promote the growth of beneficial bacteria in the gut. Increased consumption of dietary fiber and whole grains is helpful in normalizing the symbiosis of the gut micro biota and can improve gut micro biota interactions in obesity and other metabolic diseases. There are differing impacts on the gut micro biota because of the diverse compositions and structures of dietary fibers and whole grains [8], some of the dietary fibers may be more beneficial against obesity than others [9].

One of the beneficial effects of fiber is to promote satiety by decreasing food intake, and also inhibits fat deposition by removing them through bile production and stool. The recommended daily intake of fiber for healthy adults is between 20 and 35 g/d [10].

Dietary fiber intake is been found to help control KCal intake as well as to reduce the risk of weight gain leading to overweight and obesity. The role of dietary fiber in energy intake is directly connected to the development of overweight and obesity and it's related to any chemical and physical properties that are connected to the satiety signal in the brain (Rolls, 1987).

The main purpose of the this study is to identify the relationship between fiber intake and obesity by examining the effects of a high fiber diet with other anthropometrical parameters such as BW, BMI and WC in 140 adults aged 20-30 years old.

2. Methodology

The study included 140 subjects (63 males and 77 females) randomly selected, aged 20-30 years old from the general population of Abu Dhabi. The study took place from Jan 2014 to May 2014. Participants with any acute or chronic disease were excluded from the study. Subjects signed a consent form and the study was approved by the ethical committee of Zayed University.

Height and weight measured by using the digital/calibrated physician scales to the nearest 0.1 cm and 100 gr, respectively. Waist circumference measured with a regulated tape to the nearest 0.1 cm. BMI was calculated by the standard formula: weight(kg)/height(m)^2. Participants were asked to consume their usual daily calorie intake and food meals and just add/or replace choices of food with high in dietary fiber (25 gr /day/women and 38gr /day/men) from a list that was given to them for a period of 1 month period. A brochure (appendix 1) was given to each person to explain the amount and types of foods high in fiber. Data were analyzed using Microsoft EXCEL program and SPSS program. Statistically significant difference was set at $P < 0.05$.

3. Results

Table 1 displays the main characteristics of the women subjects before and after fiber intervention. A clinical small reduction was noted for body weight BMI and WC. However these changes were not significantly important.

Similarly, Table 2 shows the changes for male subjects. The mean and SD for weight, BMI, and waist for men before and after changes their diet. The weight mean before was 98.64 and it decreased to 97.54 and SD was 14.13 and declined to 14.61. The waist mean reduced by 0.28 and SD decreased by 0.22 from (mean ± SD) 96.4 ± 6.93 to 96.12 ± 6.71.

The Z test was used for analysis of pre and post intervention data for both females and males. The independent sample z test was used for comparison the results between the intervention of before and after one month of high intake of Fiber in the same group of female and male.

Parameter		Minimum	Maximum	Mean	SD	Z Value	P value
Age (year)	Before	20	30	24.77	2.75	-	-
	After	20	30	24.77	2.75		
Height	Before	153	174	162.78	3.88	-	-
	After	153	174	162.78	3.88		
Weight	Before	65.5	126	88.27	14.13	0.5607	
	After	63.9	123.6	87	13.98		0.575
BMI	Before	25	47	33.35	5.5	0.5332	
	After	24	46	32.88	5.44		0.5939
Waist	Before	80	111	94.05	7.28	0.2335	
	After	80	110	93.78	7.07		0.81537

TABLE 1: Characteristics of female subjects (n = 77) before and after intervention.

Parameter		Minimum	Maximum	Mean	SD	Z Value	P value
Age (year)	Before	20	30	25.57	3.25	-	-
	After	20	30	25.57	3.25		
Height	Before	165	184	175.59	4.15	-	-
	After	165	184	175.59	4.15		
Weight	Before	79.2	143	98.64	14.7	0.4213	
	After	77.8	140	97.54	14.61		0.6735
BMI	Before	25	48	32.06	5.12	0.3966	
	After	25	47	31.7	5.07		0.6917
Waist	Before	85	119	96.4	6.93	0.2303	
	After	85	117	96.12	6.71		0.8179

TABLE 2: Characteristics of Male subjects (n = 63) before and after intervention.

		Mean	Mean difference%	95% CI (LL,UL)	SD
Weight	Before	88.27	1.45	(-12.68),15.58	14.13
	After	87		(-12.53),15.43	13.98
BMI	Before	33.35	1.42	(-4.08),7.81	5.5
	After	32.88		(-4.02),6.86	5.44
Waist	Before	94.05	0.29	(-6.99), 7.57	7.28
	After	93.78		(-6.78),7.36	7.07

TABLE 3: % Changes on Body Weight among **Female**.

		Mean	Mean difference%	95% CI (LL,UL)	SD
Weight	Before	98.64	1.12	(-13.58),15.82	14.7
	After	97.54		(-13.49),15.73	14.61
BMI	Before	32.04	1.07	(-4.05),6.19	5.12
	After	31.7		(-4.00),6.14	5.07
Waist	Before	96.4	0.29	(-6.64), 7.22	6.93
	After	96.12		(-6.42),7.00	6.71

TABLE 4: % Changes on Body Weight among **Male**.

A small reduction is observed in weight of females as shown in (Table 3) by 1.45% from (mean ± SD) 88.27 ± 14.13 to 87.00 ± 13.98, (95% CI: -12.68 to 15.98; where the value of P is > than 0.05 so the result is not significant. And, BMI also reduced as shown (Table 3) by 0.29% from (mean ± SD) 33.35 ± 5.5 to 32.88 ± 5.44.

A small drop was also observed for males in weight as shown in (Table 4) by 1.12% from (mean ± SD) 98.64 ± 14.7 to 97.54 ± 14.61, (95% CI: -13.58 to 15.82; where the value of P > 0.05 so the result is not significant), as wall as for BMI as observed (in the Table 4) by 1.07% from (mean ± SD) 32.04 ± 5.12 to 31.70 ± 5.07. Where the value of p, the result is not significant at p > than 0.05

A small decrease in waist as shown (in Table 4) by 0.29% from (mean ± SD) 96.4 ± 6.93 (95% CI: (-6.34), to 7.22, where the value of p > 0.05. So the null hypothesis is rejected.

4. Discussion

The results show that the intake of 25 g/ day fiber for women and 38 g/ day for men during one month resulted in insignificant weight, BMI, and waist percentage reduction (P > 0.05). Fiber is always associated inversely with body fat and body weight. Furthermore, fiber intake is also inversely associated with BMI at different levels of heavy fat intake after collaborating for confounding aspects [12].

In this study 140 participants consumed diet high in dietary fiber and the effects on weight, BMI, and waist were considered among these participants. There are equivocal results from previous studies. Body weight reduction is usually described by satiety or decreased intake of food after eating fibrous food. The results explain that the use of fiber with vegetables, fruits, whole grains, and legumes, and throughout the life is considered to be very crucial. There are different mechanisms which have been suggested in order to make a clear idea about the usage of fiber aids for the purpose of weight reduction and decreasing absorption of macronutrients. Many mechanisms have been suggested for how fiber aids in weight management, decreasing absorption of macronutrients, including promoting satiation and changing secretion of specific hormones [13].

The sample was collected from different age groups and examined their food intake in different time intervals.

The results of study support the fat mass regulation and body weight, which are produced due to interplay of different factors which includes peripheral sensation stimuli, central nervous circuits, chemical and mechanical satiation signals rising in the afferent vagal input and tract of gastrointestinal. The study focuses on the trend of obesity in different age groups [13].

Another study shows that today's diet has changed as it is becoming more common, for example, food from takeaway establishments; also, the intake of high-fat products, and animal calorie sweeteners with low consumption of fiber from fruits, vegetables or whole grains creating a substantial problem. Obesity is the balance between excessive food energy intake and expenditure, from infromation above, the only way to prevent or treat obesity is to reduce caloric intake and increases energy expenditure through physical activity. It decreases the size of portions at each meal as an X variable and increase physical activity as a variable Y to make the equation lean more towards a healthy life [14].

Another study, in support of this study results shows that the dietary fiber food or is a powerful ally to prevent or tackle obesity. One of the recommendations made in relation to the daily diet, is precisely replace foods high in fat and sugar for those high in dietary fiber, which are obtained from the consumption of whole fruits, leafy vegetables, whole grains, beans unstrained and meats. Foods high in fiber also have the ability to hold water and require more chewing and salivation, which is why they cause satiety The fiber produces a reduction of gastric emptying and delayed so desires to consume food [15].

According to one more study, it is recommended to consume daily foods rich in dietary fiber, distributed in different meals, with the ingestion of fruits and vegetables along with their skins, where possible, because it is where the greatest amount of fiber is stored, and also consume citrus fruits with skins and/or take the juices without straining [16].

Limitation of the study included the short time period for the intervention as well as the absence of additional information of the subjects such as genetics, dietary habits and physical activity levels. Nevertheless, this study may have some future clinical benefits in Body Weight and Waist Circumference reduction when a high fiber diet is consumed.

5. Conclusions

Even though there was no statistically significantly difference between a high fiber diet and Body Weight, BMI and Wiast Circumference, the small clinical decreases in those parameters may be a promising future indication to continue consuming a diet high in fiber. Additionally, people will continue benefit of consuming a diet high in fiber in order to avoid future medical health problems, such as, cancer, diabetes type 2, cardiovascular diseases and metabolic syndrome.

References

[1] A. S. Beller, "Fat Thin: A Natural History of Obesity," *Farrar, Straus & Giroux*, 1977.

[2] S. Wild, G. Roglic, A. Green, R. Sicree, and H. King, "Global prevalence of diabetes: estimates for the year 2000 and projections for 2030," *Diabetes Care*, vol. 27, no. 5, pp. 1047–1053, 2004.

[3] C. L. Ogden, M. D. Carroll, B. K. Kit, and K. M. Flegal, "Prevalence of childhood and adult obesity in the United States, 2011-2012," *The Journal of the American Medical Association*, vol. 311, no. 8, pp. 806–814, 2014.

[4] M. Saberi, *UAE the fifth most obese country in the world*, Gulf News, Dubai, 2012.

[5] A. O. Musaiger, M. Al-Mannai, R. Tayyem et al., "Prevalence of overweight and obesity among adolescents in seven Arab Countries: A cross-cultural study," *Journal of Obesity*, vol. 2012, Article ID 981390, 2012.

[6] M. Malik and A. Bakir, "Prevalence of overweight and obesity among children in the United Arab Emirates," *Obesity Reviews*, vol. 8, no. 1, pp. 15–20, 2007.

[7] A. Kerkadi, N. Abo-Elnaga, and W. Ibrahim, "Prevalence of overweight and associated risk factors among primary female school children in Al-Ain city, United Arab Emirates," *Emirates Journal of Food and Agriculture*, vol. 17, no. 1, pp. 43–56, 2005.

[8] J. Snart, R. Bibiloni, T. Grayson et al., "Supplementation of the diet with high-viscosity beta-glucan results in enrichment for lactobacilli in the rat cecum," *Applied and Environmental Microbiology*, vol. 72, no. 3, pp. 1925–1931, 2006.

[9] P. Bjoerntorp, "Dietary fiber and obesity. Proceedings of a Satellite Symposium to the second Washington Symposium on Dietary Fibers," Washington, DC, USA, 1984.

[10] S. M. Pilch, "Effect of one week of fibre supplementation on hunger and satiety ratings and energy intake," in *Physiological Effects and Health Consequences of Dietary Fiber. Life Sciences Research Office*, pp. 149–157, MD, Bethesda, 1987.

[11] B. J. Rolls, "Effects of food quality, quantity, and variety on intake," in *Not Eating Enough*, B. M. Marriott, Ed., pp. 203–215, National Academy Press, Washington, DC, 1995.

[12] S. S. Gropper and P. B. Acosta, "Brief communication: The therapeutic effect of fiber in treating obesity," *Journal of the American College of Nutrition*, vol. 6, no. 6, pp. 533–535, 1987.

[13] J. L. Slavin, "Dietary fiber and body weight," *Nutrition Journal* , vol. 21, no. 3, pp. 411–418, 2005.

[14] S. Liu, WC. Willet, JE. Manson, Hu. FB, B. Rosner, and G. Colditz, "Relation between changes in intakes of dietary fiber and grain products and changes in weight and development of obesity among middleaged women," *Am J Clin Nutr*, vol. 78, no. 5, pp. 920–927, 2003.

[15] S. B. Roberts and M. B. Heyman, "Dietary composition and obesity: do we need to look beyond dietary fat," *J Nutr*, pp. 130–267S, 2000.

[16] B. J. Rolls, J. A. Ello-Martin, and B. C. Tohill, "What Can Intervention Studies Tell Us about the Relationship between Fruit and Vegetable Consumption and Weight Management?" *Nutrition Reviews*, vol. 62, no. 1, pp. 1–17, 2004.

16

Does Caffeine Enhance Athletic Performance?

Marcou Juliana and Savva Rafaella-Maria

Department of Life and Health Sciences, University of Nicosia, Nicosia, Cyprus

Corresponding Author: Savva Rafaella-Maria; email: cerdida22@hotmail.com

Abstract

Aim: A plethora of studies have been conducted to examine the effect of caffeine on athletic performance, with conflicting results. The purpose of the study is to investigate the effects of caffeine on muscle activity, physical training, competitive sports events and short-term physical activity.

Methods: For the purpose of the research, a literature review was conducted to determine the optimal dosage of caffeine for athletes, and collected scientific evidence about the caffeine's effect on athletic endurance. The inclusion criteria contain original articles with primary data collection, both quantitative and qualitative published research studies, and studies with athletic subjects. The exclusion criteria comprises review articles without outcome data, incorrect study type, studies with < 10 subjects, and studies with physical inactive subjects.

Results: An issue for dietitians and other sports medicine personnel is that all recommend that exercising athletes should avoid the use of caffeine because it is a diuretic, and that it may exacerbate dehydration and hyperthermia. Evidence indicates that consuming a moderate level of caffeine results in a mild increase of urine production. There is no evidence suggesting that moderate caffeine intake (<456 mg) induces chronic dehydration or negatively affects exercise performance. In addition, pre-exercise feeding may significantly affect plasma caffeine concentrations and the potential for caffeine to improve performance. On the other hand, recent studies suggest that caffeine might indeed have ergogenic potential in endurance events. Also, reports concerning caffeine's effect on VO2 max and exercise performance during incremental exercise are not in agreement. However, few caffeine studies have been published to include cognitive and physiologic considerations for the athlete. Furthermore, the effects of different doses of caffeine play important role on endurance. In addition, exercise time to exhaustion seems to be different between users and nonusers with the ergogenic effect being greater and lasting longer in nonusers.

Conclusion: Caffeine consumption may enhance athletic endurance, based on strong evidence, but further research needs to be conducted. High caffeine doses than the optimal, 3-6 mg/kg, before exercise does not confer any additional improvement in athletic performance. Additional, higher caffeine doses may cause side effects in athletes.

Keywords: Caffeine; Exercise; Athletic performance; Sports nutrition

1. Introduction

Caffeine is a pharmacological compound that is extracted on a large scale from the plant coffee Arabica, which originated in Ethiopia. Caffeine and the related substances, theophylline and theobromine, are components of food and drinks, and for most people these substances are part of their daily diet (table 1). Caffeine may be the most prevalent stimulant drug in world. The use is not prohibited for athletes, with a maximum allowable concentration 12 mg/L of urine (International Olympic Committee).

A plethora of studies have been conducted to examine the effect of caffeine on athletic performance, with conflicting results. The fact that caffeine affects the central nervous system, adipose tissue and skeletal muscle, initially led to the hypothesis that caffeine can affect athletic performance. Strong evidence shows that caffeine enhances endurance and provide improvement of performance in a wide range of different physical exercises: short duration, high-intensity events (1-5 minutes), prolonged high-intensity events (20-60 minutes), endurance events (>90 minutes), ultra-endurance events (>4 hours) and prolonged intermittent sprint events (team sports). Caffeine may enhance contractile force in skeletal muscle during submaximal contraction and increase the athlete's threshold for pain or perceived exertion, which could result in longer training sessions [33]. As a powerful antioxidant, caffeine can help combat the muscle damage caused by exercise [39].

For many years, research into caffeine's energy-boosting effects was focused on examining its effects on endurance exercise. As a result, a great deal of data was collected incontrovertibly establishing that caffeine has ergogenic power in exercise situations in which fatigue occurs in 30 to 60 minutes [39]. Caffeine may enhance endurance performance by increasing the release of adrenaline into the blood stimulating the release of free fatty acids from fat tissue and skeletal muscle. Caffeine also does not alter exercise metabolism, and therefore, it appears that alterations in muscle metabolism alone cannot fully explain the ergogenic effect of caffeine during endurance exercise.

Short-term exercise has received much less attention. In the last two decades, researchers have deliberated the effects of caffeine on short-term exercise with progressive work tests, in which athletes undertake high-intensity exercise that results in rapid exhaustion. Researches suggest that caffeine ingestion improves performance during short-term exercise, lasting approximately 5 minute at 90-100 % of maximal oxygen uptake. This exercise intensity requires maximal provision of energy from both aerobic and anaerobic systems. The reasons for the performance improvement may be direct positive effect of caffeine on muscle anaerobic energy provision and contraction or a central nervous component related to the sensation of effort, leading

Food/Drink	Portion	Caffeine (mg/cup)
Filter coffee	200 ml	90
Espresso	60 ml	80
Tea	220 ml	40–60
Plain chocolate	50 g	20–25
Milk chocolate	50 g	~10
Soft Drinks (coca cola, etc.)	355 ml	40
Energy Drink	250 ml	~80

TABLE 1: EFSA, 2015.

to a reduction in perception of effort during exercise and therefore influencing the motivational factors to sustain effort during exercise [29].

Studies on caffeine use in strength training, is less prevalent than in endurance training. However, evidence strongly suggests that caffeine has direct effects on the strength of muscle performance that are independent of caffeine's metabolic effects. According to Graham [19], caffeine may increase strength by changing the environments of active muscles in a way that can "facilitate force production" by the muscle's cells.

Additionally, it is well known that caffeine use has several side effects. Blood pressure is increased both at rest and during exercise, heart rate is increased, gastrointestinal distress can occur and insomnia can result [33]. At high levels, caffeine has the potential to cause impairments or alterations in fine motor skills and techniques, and it can interfere with recovery and sleep patterns, more likely in athletes who are not regular caffeine users. Since dehydration is a concern of every athlete, series of studies occur for decades, in order to examine the possible effect of caffeine on dehydration. For several years, athletes avoid consumed caffeine, because of the myth that caffeine may cause dehydration [39]. In the past few years, researchers have proven that caffeine does not dehydrate athletic people and has no diuretic effects at all on people who exercise. There is no evidence that caffeine ingestion before exercise leads to dehydration, or other side effects such as ion imbalance and stomach irritation. However, athletes must consume caffeine in the optimal dose 3-6 mg/kg, in order to avoid side effects. In addition, handful of studies has failed to find any further improvement on athletic performance, in very high doses.

The purpose of the study is to investigate the effects of caffeine to muscle activity, physical training, competitive sports events and short-term physical activity. The optimal dose of caffeine for athletes and possible side effects, will be also discussed.

For the purpose of the research, a literature review was conducted to determine the optimal dosage of caffeine for athletes and collect scientific evidence about the caffeine's effect on athletic endurance. The literature search held through electronic databases and articles in scientific journals such as Sports Medicine and Journal of Medicine and Science in Sports, etc. The main databases used were: PubMed, World Health Organization (WHO), International Olympic Committee (IOC) and National Center for Biotechnology Information (NCBI). The following words – keys, used during the search: caffeine, athletes, performance, endurance, strength, side effects, dosage, exercise.

The inclusion criteria of the literature review contain original articles with primary data collection, both quantitative and qualitative research published studies, and studies with athletic subjects. The language of publication was narrowed to English and publication date from November 2015, with no longer limit date was chosen. The exclusion criteria comprise review articles without outcome data, incorrect study type, studies with < 10 subjects, and studies with physical inactive subjects.

2. Discussion

An issue for dietitians, exercise physiologists, athletic trainers, and other sports medicine personnel all recommend that exercising athletes should avoid the use of caffeine because it is a diuretic, and it may exacerbate dehydration and hyperthermia. Evidence indicates that consuming a moderate level of caffeine results in a mild increase of urine production. Although this diuresis may (240-642 mg of caffeine) or may not (<240 mg) be significantly greater than a control fluid (0 mg of caffeine), there is no evidence suggesting that moderate caffeine intake (<456 mg) induces chronic dehydration or negatively affects exercise performance, temperature regulation, and circulatory strain in a hot environment. Caffeinated fluids contribute to the daily human water requirement in a manner that is similar to pure water. It is possible that urinary Na+, but less likely that urinary K+, excretion is increased somewhat by caffeine consumption. However, an affluent Western diet provides Na+ and K+ in amounts that exceed these losses. Furthermore, no evidence supports the contention that caffeine increases heat storage during exercise or that caffeine affects exercise performance in a hot environment negatively. Finally, not enough research where done about the efficacy of caffeine administration regarding large doses of caffeine (>600 mg) that are consumed at one time and differences between modes of caffeine delivery, for instance via capsules, tablets, coffee, tea, soft drinks, sport drinks, and solid food [25].

The enhanced endurance performance observed in athletes consuming coffee containing 330 mg of caffeine 60 minutes before the exercise had similar effects of caffeine on lipolysis and has positive influence on nerve impulse transmission [8]. Skinner, T. L., et al, [34] agrees that individual characteristics need to be considered when administering caffeine for performance enhancement. In addition, pre-exercise feeding may significantly affect plasma caffeine concentrations and the potential for caffeine to improve performance. On the other hand, recent studies suggest that caffeine might indeed have ergogenic potential in endurance events (e.g. marathon running). It is hypothesized that it is related to the increased availability of free fatty acids for muscle metabolism, which has a glycogen-sparing effect. Also, reports concerning caffeine's effect on $\dot{V}O_2$ max and exercise performance during incremental exercise are not in agreement [31].

An interesting study, Lorino, A. J. [26], suggested that a 6 mg [middle dot] kg-1 dose of caffeine does not impact agility as measured by the proagility run test or power output as measured by the 30-second Wingate test in recreationally active young adult males who are not habituated to caffeine.

An important aspect is the ergogenic effect of caffeine on athletic performance that has been discussed in many studies. However, few caffeine studies have been published to include cognitive and physiologic considerations for the athlete. The following practical recommendations consider the global effects of caffeine on the body resulted that lower doses can be as effective as higher doses during exercise performance without any negative coincidence after a period of cessation, restarting caffeine intake at a low amount before exercise performance can provide the same ergogenic effects as acute intake. Basically, caffeine can be taken gradually at low doses to avoid tolerance during the course of 3 or 4 days, just before intense training to sustain exercise intensity and caffeine can improve cognitive aspects of performance, such as concentration, for instance when an athlete has not slept well. [35]. A similar recent study was done and stated that, lower caffeine doses (≤3 mg/kg bm, ~200 mg) taken before exercise increases athletic performance. Low caffeine doses do not alter exercise-induced changes in peripheral whole-body responses to exercise and are associated with few side effects. Low doses of caffeine (~200 mg) have also been shown to improve awareness, alertness and mood and improve cognitive processes during and following strenuous exercise. Therefore, the ergogenic effect of low caffeine doses appears to result from alterations in the central nervous system [25].

Many studies indicate that, during aerobic exercise a nutritionally-enriched coffee beverage appears to enhance time to exhaustion, whereas, it does not provide an ergogenic benefit during anaerobic exercise [21].

Furthermore, the effects of different doses of caffeine play important role on endurance cycling time trial performance. Desbrow, B. [10] concluded that a caffeine dose of 3 mg·kg−1 body mass appears to improve cycling performance in well-trained and familiarized athletes. Whereas, doubling the dose of caffeine to 6 mg·kg−1 body mass does not confer any additional improvements in performance. A similar came to the same conclusion that high caffeine dose had the greatest effect on epinephrine and blood-borne metabolites yet had the least effect on performance. While, low caffeine dose had little or no effect on epinephrine and metabolites but did have an ergogenic effect. These results are not compatible with the traditional theory that caffeine mediates its ergogenic effect via enhanced catecholamines [17].

As stated before, caffeine is a common substance used by most athletes, and it is now found as well in many new products, including energy drinks, sport gels, alcoholic beverages and diet aids. It can be a powerful ergogenic aid at levels that are considerably lower than the acceptable levels of the International Olympic Committee and could be beneficial in training and in competition. Caffeine does not improve maximal oxygen capacity directly, but could permit the athlete to train at a greater power output and train longer time. It is indicated that intake of caffeine increase speed and power output in simulated race conditions. These effects have been found in activities that last as little as 60 seconds or as long as 2 hours. Not enough research was done in order to see if caffeine affects the strength of the athlete. However, a study claimed that there was no effect on maximal ability, but enhanced endurance or resistance to fatigue. Also, not further research was done to see if caffeine ingestion before exercise leads to dehydration, ion imbalance, or any other adverse effects. Due to that ingestion of caffeine as coffee appears to be ineffective compared to doping with pure caffeine. It appears that male and female athletes have similar caffeine pharmacokinetics, for instance a given dose of caffeine, the time course and absolute plasma concentrations of caffeine and its metabolites are the same. So, exercise or dehydration does not affect caffeine pharmacokinetics. Limited studies suggest that caffeine non-users and users respond similarly and that withdrawal from caffeine may not be important [19].

In addition to this, exercise time to exhaustion seems to be different between users and nonusers with the ergogenic effect being greater and lasting longer in nonusers, according to Bell & McLellan [4]. For the nonusers (8 subjects), exercise times 1, 3, and 6 h after caffeine ingestion, <50 mg caffeine/day were significantly greater. But, for caffeine users (13 subjects), exercise times 1, 3, and 6 h after caffeine ingestion (>300 mg caffeine/day) were respectively. Only exercise times 1 and 3 h after drug ingestion were significantly greater. The study concluded that 5 mg/kg dose of caffeine were greater in the nonusers compared with the users.

A lot of studies aimed to see the effect of caffeine on exercise performance in habitual caffeine users. A study suggested that habitually high caffeine users acquire a tolerance to caffeine, which reduces its effects during prolonged exercise. Furthermore, to magnify the effect of caffeine, habitual users should withdraw from caffeine use for about 4 days [15].

Another study aimed was to examine the effects of caffeine ingestion on exercise performance at low and high altitudes. The effect of caffeine on exercise time over a specified distance (approx. 21 km) was investigated in well-trained cross-country skiers (14 subjects) both at low (300 m above sea level) and high (2900 m above sea level) altitudes. Each subject participated in two races at both altitudes - one after caffeine ingestion (6 mg/kg body weight) and one after placebo on a double-blind basis. They concluded that caffeine induces had an increased in performance capacity for cross-country skiers at low altitudes [5].

Sung, et al., [37] present study examined the effects of caffeine on blood pressure regulation in hypertensive men during exercise. Twenty unmedicated, mild hypertensives (HT, BP = 140/90 to 160/105 mm Hg) and 12 age-matched, normotensives (NT, BP < 130/80 mm Hg) performed 30 min of extended bicycle exercise following a single dose of caffeine (3.3 mg/kg, equivalent to 2 to 3 cups of coffee) and placebo in a double-blind, cross-over design. He claimed that during exercise, heart rate was greater on caffeine day than placebo day in hypertensives only. Systolic blood pressure was consistently elevated on caffeine day compared to placebo day in both groups. Diastolic blood pressure was elevated in hypertensives for 30 min of exercise on caffeine day, but this disappeared at 15 min of exercise in normotensives. As a result, rate-pressure products were significantly higher on caffeine days in hypertensives at post drug and during exercise. On caffeine day, 7 hypertensives and 1 normotensive showed an excessive blood pressure response during exercise. This study assumed that caffeine has significant hemodynamic effects on mild hypertensives at rest and during exercise. The increased rate-pressure products following caffeine during exercise place a greater workload on the heart, and abstinence from caffeine, especially before exercise, may be effective for persons with hypertension.

3. Conclusion

The purpose of the study was to collect information on caffeine's benefits to muscle activity, physical training, competitive sports events and short-term physical activity, which aims to examine the hypothesis that caffeine enhance athlete's endurance. It appears that, caffeine consumption may enhance athletic endurance in both short duration activities and long endurance exercises, based on strong evidence. As the result seems controversial on ergogenic effect on caffeine, further research needs to be conducted. The optimal dose of caffeine for athletes and possible side effects were considered during the research. High caffeine doses than the optimal, 3-6 mg/kg, before exercise does not confer any additional improvement in athletic performance. Additional, higher caffeine doses may cause side effects in athletes, such as increased blood pressure and heart rate.

References

[1] L. E. Armstrong, D. J. Casa, C. M. Maresh, and M. S. Ganio, "Caffeine, fluid-electrolyte balance, temperature regulation, and exercise-heat tolerance," *Exercise and Sport Sciences Reviews*, vol. 35, no. 3, pp. 135–140, 2007.

[2] J. J. Barone and H. R. Roberts, "Caffeine consumption," *Food and Chemical Toxicology*, vol. 34, no. 1, pp. 119–129, 1996.

[3] D. S. Battram, T. E. Graham, E. A. Richter, and F. Dela, "The effect of caffeine on glucose kinetics in humans-influence of adrenaline," *The Journal of Physiology*, vol. 569, no. 1, pp. 347–355, 2005.

[4] D. G. Bell and T. M. McLellan, "Exercise endurance 1, 3, and 6 h after caffeine ingestion in caffeine users and nonusers," *Journal of Applied Physiology*, vol. 93, no. 4, pp. 1227–1234, 2002.

[5] B. Berglund and P. Hemmingsson, "Effects of caffeine ingestion on exercise performance at low and high altitudes in cross-country skiers," *International Journal of Sports Medicine*, vol. 3, no. 4, pp. 234–236, 1982.

[6] D. Bracco, J.-M. Ferrarra, M. J. Arnaud, E. Jequier, and Y. Schutz, "Effects of caffeine on energy metabolism, heart rate, and methylxanthine metabolism in lean and obese women," *American Journal of Physiology-Endocrinology and Metabolism*, vol. 269, no. 4, pp. E671–E678, 1995.

[7] L. M. Burke, "Caffeine and sports performance," *Applied Physiology, Nutrition, and Metabolism*, vol. 33, no. 6, pp. 1319–1334, 2008.

[8] D. L. Costill, G. P. Dalsky, and W. J. Fink, "Effects of caffeine ingestion on metabolism and exercise performance," *Medicine & Science in Sports & Exercise*, vol. 10, no. 3, pp. 155–158, 1978.

[9] J. K. Davis and J. M. Green, "Caffeine and anaerobic performance: ergogenic value and mechanisms of action," *Sports Medicine*, vol. 39, no. 10, pp. 813–832, 2009.

[10] B. Desbrow, C. Biddulph, B. Devlin, G. D. Grant, S. Anoopkumar-Dukie, and M. D. Leveritt, "The effects of different doses of caffeine on endurance cycling time trial performance," *Journal of Sports Sciences*, vol. 30, no. 2, pp. 115–120, 2012.

[11] S. L. Dodd, E. Brooks, S. K. Powers, and R. Tulley, "The effects of caffeine on graded exercise performance in caffeine naive versus habituated subjects," *European Journal of Applied Physiology*, vol. 62, no. 6, pp. 424–429, 1991.

[12] M. Doherty and P. M. Smith, "Effects of caffeine ingestion on rating of perceived exertion during and after exercise: A meta-analysis," *Scandinavian Journal of Medicine & Science in Sports*, vol. 15, no. 2, pp. 69–78, 2005.

[13] EFSA. Caffeine. [online] Available from http://www.efsa.europa.eu/sites/default/files/corporate_publications/files/efsaexplainscaffeine150527.pdf.

[14] M. M. Fisher, "The Effect of Resistance Exercise on Recovery Blood Pressure in Normotensive and Borderline Hypertensive Women," *The Journal of Strength and Conditioning Research*, vol. 15, no. 2, pp. 210–216, 2001.

[15] S. M. Fisher, R. G. McMurray, M. Berry, M. H. Mar, and W. A. Forsythe, "Influence of caffeine on exercise performance in habitual caffeine users," *International Journal of Sports Medicine*, vol. 7, no. 5, pp. 276–280, 1986.

[16] T. E. Graham and L. L. Spriet, "Caffeine and Exercise Performance," in *Sport Science Exchange*, vol. 9, p. 60, Sport Science Exchange, 1996.

[17] T. E. Graham and L. L. Spriet, "Metabolic, catecholamine, and exercise performance responses to various doses of caffeine," *Journal of Applied Physiology*, vol. 78, no. 3, pp. 867–874, 1995.

[18] T. E. Graham, "Caffeine and exercise metabolism, endurance and performance," *Sports Medicine*, vol. 31, no. 11, pp. 785–807, 2012.

[19] T. E. Graham, "Caffeine and exercise metabolism, endurance and performance," *Sports Medicine*, vol. 31, no. 11, pp. 785–807, 2001.

[20] C. R. Hendrix, T. J. Housh, M. Mielke et al., "Acute effects of a caffeine-containing supplement on bench press and leg extension strength and time to exhaustion during cycle ergometry," *The Journal of Strength and Conditioning Research*, vol. 24, no. 3, pp. 859–865, 2010.

[21] J. R. Hoffman, J. I. E. Kang, N. A. Ratamess, P. F. Jennings, G. T. Mangine, and A. D. Faigenbaum, "Effect of nutritionally enriched coffee consumption on aerobic and anaerobic exercise performance," *The Journal of Strength and Conditioning Research*, vol. 21, no. 2, pp. 456–459, 2007.

[22] J. L. Ivy, D. L. Costill, W. J. Fink, and R. W. Lower1, "Influence of caffeine and carbohydrate feedings on endurance performance," *Medicine & Science in Sports & Exercise*, vol. 11, no. 1, pp. 6–11, 1979.

[23] B. H. Jacobson, M. D. Weber, L. Claypool, and L. E. Hunt, "Effect of caffeine on maximal strength and power in elite male athletes," *British Journal of Sports Medicine*, vol. 26, no. 4, pp. 276–280, 1992.

[24] L. A. Kaminsky, C. A. Martin, and M. H. Whaley, "Caffeine consumption habits do not influence the exercise blood pressure response following caffeine ingestion," *The Journal of Sports Medicine and Physical Fitness* , vol. 38, no. 1, pp. 53–58, 1998.

[25] L. L. Spriet, "Exercise and Sport Performance with Low Doses of Caffeine," *Sports Medicine*, vol. 44, pp. 175–184, 2014.

[26] A. J. Lorino, L. K. Lloyd, S. H. Crixell, and J. L. Walker, "The effects of caffeine on athletic agility," *The Journal of Strength and Conditioning Research*, vol. 20, no. 4, pp. 851–854, 2006.

[27] B. R. MacIntosh and B. M. Wright, "Caffeine ingestion and performance of a 1,500-metre swim.," *Canadian journal of applied physiology = Revue canadienne de physiologie appliquée*, vol. 20, no. 2, pp. 168–177, 1995.

[28] S. R. McClaran and T. J. Wetter, "Low doses of caffeine reduce heart rate during submaximal cycle ergometry," *Journal of the International Society of Sports Nutrition*, vol. 4, article no. 11, 2007.

[29] R. Meeusen, B. Roelands, and L. L. Spriet, "Caffeine, exercise and the brain," *Nestle Nutrition Institute Workshop Series*, vol. 76, pp. 1–12, 2013.

[30] W. J. Pasman, M. A. Van Baak, A. E. Jeukendrup, and A. De Haan, "The effect of different dosages of caffeine on endurance performance time," *International Journal of Sports Medicine*, vol. 16, no. 4, pp. 225–230, 1995.

[31] S. K. Powers and S. Dodd, "Caffeine and Endurance Performance," *Sports Medicine*, vol. 2, no. 3, pp. 165–174, 1985.

[32] T. Richardson, A. Rozkovec, P. Thomas, J. Ryder, C. Meckes, and D. Kerr, "Influence of Caffeine on Heart Rate Variability in Patients with Long-Standing Type 1 Diabetes," *Diabetes Care*, vol. 27, no. 5, pp. 1127–1131, 2004.

[33] CA. Rosenbloom and EJ. Coleman, "Sports Nutrition: A Practice," in *Manual for Professionals, Chicago, IL: Academy of Nutrition and Dietetics*, Academy of Nutrition and Dietetics, IL, 5th edition, 2015.

[34] T. L. Skinner, D. G. Jenkins, J. S. Coombes, D. R. Taaffe, and M. D. Leveritt, "Dose response of caffeine on 2000-m rowing performance," *Medicine & Science in Sports & Exercise*, vol. 42, no. 3, pp. 571–576, 2010.

[35] B. Sökmen, L. E. Armstrong, W. J. Kraemer et al., "Caffeine use in sports: considerations for the athlete," *The Journal of Strength and Conditioning Research*, vol. 22, no. 3, pp. 978–986, 2008.

[36] T. E. Graham and L. L. Spriet, "Performance and metabolic responses to a high caffeine dose during prolonged exercise," *Journal of Applied Physiology*, vol. 71, no. 6, pp. 2292–2298, 1991.

[37] B. H. Sung, W. R. Lovallo, T. Whitsett, and M. F. Wilson, "Caffeine elevates blood pressure response to exercise in mild hypertensive men," *American Journal of Hypertension*, vol. 8, no. 12, pp. 1184–1188, 1995.

[38] T. J. Vandenbogaerde and W. G. Hopkins, "Monitoring acute effects on athletic performance with mixed linear modeling," *Medicine & Science in Sports & Exercise*, vol. 42, no. 7, pp. 1339–1344, 2010.

[39] B. A. Weinberg and B. K. Bealer, *The Caffeine Advantage*, The Free Press, New York, 2002.

[40] J. Weir, T. D. Noakes, K. Myburgh, and B. Adams, "A high carbohydrate diet negates the metabolic effects of caffeine during exercise," *Medicine & Science in Sports & Exercise*, vol. 19, no. 2, pp. 100–105, 1987.

17

Association of Beverage Consumption with Obesity in Healthy Adults

Sirine Maher Zahran

Department of Natural Sciences and Public Health, Zayed University, Abu Dhabi, UAE

Corresponding Author: Sirine Maher Zahran; email:s_mz9@hotmail.com

Abstract

Background: The increased consumption of sugar-sweetened beverages (SSBs) has been found to be an important contributor of calories in the diet. Whether there is an association between the increased consumption of SSBs and the high rates of overweight and obesity is still questionable. The objective of this study was to examine the relationship of weight status and beverages consumed of adults in a residential compound in Abu Dhabi.

Methods: Forty nine out of 65 residents form Al Reef Villas in Abu Dhabi agreed to participate in the study. Initial assessments including beverages frequency questionnaire and anthropometry measurements were completed for all participants. Participants who were identified as high beverages consumers were invited to a one-month intervention aiming to limit their beverages consumption. A final assessment was completed for all high consumers of beverages at the end of the one-month intervention.

Results: 55% of the subjects were overweight or obese, and 51% had abdominal obesity. 73% consumed 100% fruit juices with no added sugar, 65% consumed soft drinks, and 60 % consumed plain milk and milk products. The majority (69%) consumed tea beverages rather than coffee beverages. There was no association between weight & beverages consumption. The mean energy percentage from beverages was 14.2 (±11.1) among all participants. 53% were considered high consumers of beverages and 47% (n = 23) were considered low consumers of beverages. The one-month intervention showed a significant decrease in % of calories from beverages and weight in the overweight & obese intervention group ($p < 0.001$ and $p < 0.05$) respectively.

Conclusion: This study highlighted major health problems in Abu Dhabi including high rates of overweight, obesity, and abdominal obesity. The one-month intervention was effective in reducing the energy percentage from beverages and weight of the overweight and obese participants, but no association was found in this sample between beverages consumption and overweight and obesity.

Keywords: beverages consumption, SSB, obesity, waist circumference, adults, Abu Dhabi

1. Introduction

The term "Beverages" is very broad, and several subdivisions and definitions fall beneath it. Generally, beverages are any liquids or fluids that people drink. However, there are many classifications to identify beverages. One classification is to divide beverages into alcoholic and non-alcoholic beverages depending on their alcohol content. The alcoholic beverages are drinks containing ethyl alcohol and they are produced by the fermentation of yeast, sugars, and starches. Categories of alcoholic beverages include Wine, beer, and spirits. The non-alcoholic beverages can be further subdivided into carbonated (sodas and tonic water) and non-carbonated (coffee, tea, fruit juices and fruit drinks) according to their gas (CO_2) content [7]. Second classification is to divide beverages according to their nutrient density. These include nutrient-dense beverages (water), beverages with some nutritional benefits (fruit and vegetable juices, whole milk, alcohol, and sports drinks), and nutrient-poor beverages (soft drinks and juice drinks) [17]. Another classification is to divide beverages according to their caloric and sugar content. Subcategories of this include non-caloric beverages, non-calorically sweetened beverages, natural sweet beverages, and calorically (sugar) sweetened beverages [17].

Statistics of the US population showed that 63% of adults consume sugary drinks. The current per capita consumption of sugary drinks is estimated to be 203kcal/day among adults in comparison to only 50 kcal/day in 1965 [20]. In addition, calories from SSBs increased by 60 % among the US children and the percentage of children consuming SSBs increased from 79% to 91% between 1989 and 2008. Children and youth consumed about 224 calories per day from sugary beverages in 1999 to 2004. This made up about 11% of their daily calorie intake during that period of time [21].

On the other hand, a decrease in SSBs consumption among youth and adults was observed in the United States between 1999 and 2010. The SSBS consumption decreased among youth by 68 calories/day and among adults by 45 calories/day. In 2009-2010, SSBs contributed to 8% and 6.9% of daily energy intake among youth and adults, respectively. Soda and fruit drink consumption decreased between 1999 and 2010, whereas the consumption of sports and energy drinks and sweetened coffee and teas increased [12]. In the UK, beverages accounted for 21%, 14% and 18% of energy per day for children, adolescents, and adults, respectively. Also the British children, adolescents, and adults experienced important shifts in beverages' consumption since the 1990s. The most important shifts among children and adolescents are a decrease in consumption of high-fat milk with a shift towards sodas, fruit drinks, juices, and sweetened dairy. On the other hand, consumption of dairy, sweetened tea and coffee and other energy-containing drinks decreased among adults, but alcohol and juices increased [23].

Regionally, there are limited statistics that show the consumption patterns of SSBs. However, a recent study by Basu, McKee, Galea, and Stuckler [1] studied soft drink consumption in 75 countries including the GCC. The results of it showed that soft drink consumption increased globally from 36 liters per person per year to 43.2 liters between 1997 and 2010. Furthermore, the results found that the United Arab Emirates was ranked the fifth highest country of soft drink consumption among all countries in 2010 with a consumption rate of 103.3 liters per person per year. Another study by Wen Ng et al. [24] examined the dietary patterns among Emiratis in 2009-2010. The results highlighted calories from beverages as one of the major contributors to total calories. They found that calories from beverages contributed to 8% of total calories for adult Emirati women and 14% for male Emirati children. Also the major SSBs consumption is associated with several health problems including, type 2 diabetes, metabolic syndrome, cardiovascular diseases, liver diseases, dental diseases, inadequate intake of some nutrients, and some types of cancer. The consumption of SSBs was found to have a role in the development of type 2 diabetes. SSBs contain high amounts of sugar allowing for a high glycemic load while having poor satiating properties. This affects insulin function in the body contributing to insulin resistance and β-cell dysfunction [21]. A meta-analysis by Malik et al. [14] on data from eight prospective cohort studies found that participants in the highest category of SSBs intake (most often 1–2 servings/day) had a 26% greater risk of developing type 2 diabetes than participants in the lowest category of intake (none or <1 serving/month). Similarly, a cohort study showed that women who consumed 2 to 3 SSBs per day had a 31% greater risk of developing type 2 diabetes, than women who consumed less than 1 SSB per month [2].

Another major concern in relation to SSBs is their impact on dental health especially for children. A study by Kolker et al. [13] found that African American children frequently consumed sugared drinks which were associated with the prevalence of dental caries. The results of a similar study by Warren et al. [22] done on 212 children suggested that consumption of SSBs in children up to 24 months of age is a strong and identifiable predictor of early childhood caries development. Also a related study found that high frequency of soft drink consumption and the presence of gingival plaque deposits is significantly associated with caries in low-income African-American adults [3].

The consumption of SSBs was also contributed to an inadequate intake of important nutrients including calcium, iron, folate and vitamin A by replacing milk consumption among children [19]. A study by Rodriguez-Artalejo et al. [18] found that consumption of sweetened soft drinks was associated with a lower consumption of milk among Spanish children. Another study by Harnack, Stang, and Story [8] found that US children and adolescents in the highest soft drink consumption category consumed less milk and fruit juice compared with those in the lowest consumption category.

Furthermore, some studies have shown a positive association between SSBs consumption some types of cancers including endometrial, pancreatic, and prostate cancer. A recent study found that the risk of type I endometrial cancer was 78% higher among postmenopausal women in the highest quintile of SSBs intake compared to women with zero SSBs intake [10]. Many studies have found a strong association between SSBs and overweight and obesity. A 20-year study by Mozaffarian et al. [15] has done on 120,000 men and women and found that people who increased their sugary drink consumption by one 12 Oz. serving per day gained more weight over time than people who did not change their intake. Another recent study by Basu et al., [1] has examined 75 different countries worldwide and found that a 1% rise in soft drink consumption was associated with an additional 4.8 overweight adults per 100 and 2.3 obese adults per 100.

Moreover, a study by Tol Chan [4] has investigated the association between SSBs consumption and BMI using data from the National Health and Nutrition Examination Survey 2003-2004 and concluded that average BMI was positively associated with the consumption of sugar-sweetened fruit drinks and soft drinks but not with natural fruit juices.

The main purpose of the study is to examine weight status and percentages of calories consumed from beverages of adults in a residential compound in Abu Dhabi before and after a one-month pilot intervention to decrease beverages' consumption.

2. Methodology

2.1. Participants

In this intervention study, residents from Al Reef Villas in Abu Dhabi were chosen randomly over a two weeks period during spring 2014. The study leader was passing villas every day, except for the weekend days, in the afternoon (from 4 PM – 7 PM), explaining the purpose of the visit to the first person that opens the door, and asking if he/she and/or family members are willing to take part in the study. 65 residents were invited to participate in the study. The researcher handed out written study information along with explaining the study details orally to people who were invited. In addition, written informed consent was obtained from each resident who decided to participate in the study.

2.2. Beverages Questionnaire

The assessment of the level of beverages consumption was completed using a beverages frequency questionnaire that was developed by the researcher. The questionnaire was in an online format, and was provided to participants using an iPad. Moreover, the participants were provided with cups reflecting the actual serving-sizes mentioned in the questionnaire along with putting images for the different sizes in the questionnaire to let them make accurate estimate about their beverage size. The serving-sizes of beverages reflect the common sizes, which are available at the local supermarkets and most people drink. The questionnaire was divided into a background section including demographic and health status as well as beverage sections: soft drinks, juices, energy/sport drinks, & milk drinks section, coffee and tea section, and alcohol section. The first section consisted of 7 demographical open-ended questions (name, gender, date of birth, E-mail, mobile number, villa number, and medical conditions), and a physical activity close-ended question providing options (basic everyday activities, 30 min. daily, 60 min. daily, 2≥ hours daily) from which participants selected the one that reflects their physical activity.

The second beverage section consisted of a table listing 12 different types of beverages (soft drinks, diet soft drinks, 100% fruit juices with no added sugar or syrup, fruit juices with added sugar or syrup, fruit drinks with added sugar or syrup, energy drinks, sport drinks, plain milk & milk products, flavored milk & milk products, milkshakes, smoothies), and including frequency options (Never, 1 time/week, 2-3 times/week, 4-6 times/week, 1 time/day, 2 times/day, 3 ≥ times/day) and size of the beverage that the participant drinks each time (180 ml, 250 ml, 360 ml, & 500 ml).

The third beverage section consisted of a similar table but including 10 different coffee and tea beverages (tea/herbal tea, tea/herbal tea with milk, American coffee, American coffee with milk, espresso/Turkish coffee, cappuccino, café latte, caramel latte, mocha, frappe/ Frappuccino), and there were additional options on sweetness of the beverage (no sugar, 1sugar bag/tsp, 2 sugar bags/tsps., 3 ≥ sugar bags/tsps., artificial sweetener) beside frequency and size of the beverage.

The fourth and final beverage section consisted of 7 standard servings of different types of alcoholic drinks (a can of regular beer, a glass of malt liquor, table wine, fortified wine, cordial/liqueur/aperitif, brandy, a shot of 80-proof spirits) and beside each drink there were also different options on how often and how many drinks each time (1 glass, 2 glasses, 3≥ glasses) do the participant consume that alcoholic drink. This section was optional for alcohol drinkers only.

2.3. Anthropometry Measurements

The assessment of the weight status was performed using direct measurements of height and weight to calculate BMI, and waist and hip circumferences to assess fat distribution. Weight was measured in kilograms using a calibrated digital scale, and height was measured in centimeters using a Stadiometer. All participants were asked to take off shoes when weight and height were measured. Moreover, waist and hip circumferences were measured in centimeters using a standardized measuring tape. Measurements were recorded in the questionnaire by the researcher.

3. Data Analysis

3.1. Cutoff Values

Beverage Guidance Panel [17] recommends adults to consume 10% or less of their total energy requirements from beverages. This was used as cutoff that determined if the participant was considered a high or low consumer of beverages. According to the WHO, a person with a BMI greater than or equal to 25 is considered overweight, while a person with a BMI greater than or equal to 30 is considered obese. Also the American Heart Association has defined abdominal obesity as having waist circumference ≥88 cm for women and ≥102 cm for men. These were used as cutoffs to identify overweight, obese, and abdominally obese participants.

3.2. Total Energy Requirements Calculation

Calculating the Resting Metabolic Rate (RMR) first, and further multiplying it by a physical activity coefficient provided total energy requirements for each participant. The Resting Metabolic Rate (RMR) was calculated using Mifflin-St Jeor equation as it is the preferred equation for healthy people and weight management (men: RMR = (9.99 X weight) + (6.25 X height) – (4.92 X age) + 5; women: RMR = (9.99 X weight) + (6.25 X height) – (4.92 X age) – 161).

The physical activity Coefficients was obtained from the Dietary Reference Intakes for Energy, Carbohydrate, Fiber, Fat, Fatty Acids, Cholesterol, Protein, and Amino Acids (2005). The participant's response in the health status section of the questionnaire was translated into physical activity coefficient as following:

Basic everyday activities ≈1

30 min. daily ≈1.11 (men)/1.12 (women)

60 min. daily ≈1.25 (men)/1.27 (women)

2 ≥ hours daily ≈1.48 (men)/1.45 (women)

After that, 10% of total energy requirements was calculated to identify the maximum recommended daily calories from beverages for each participant.

3.3. Calories from Beverages Calculation

Average calories of each size of each beverage in the questionnaire were calculated and used as scoring values to calculate the daily calories intake from beverages for each participant. Each participant had a scoring sheet in which the beverages that he/she drinks were listed and then calories were calculated by multiplying how often per day does the participant drink that beverage by the calories of the size he/she drinks. Then calories from SSBs, 100% fruit juices, and alcoholic beverages were summed together to calculate total calories from beverages per day for each participant. Calories from plain milk and milk products and from unsweetened tea and coffee were excluded from scoring calculations, as they are not part of the beverages that have been studied.

3.4. Intervention

After doing the assessment and calculation of daily calories from beverages and total energy requirements for all participants, those who were identified as high beverages consumers were invited to a one-month intervention by taking appointment and revisiting them. This visit involved a brief individualized discussion about the beverages of which he/she consumes a lot, how much calories and sugar do these beverages provide him/her daily, and the benefits of limiting their consumption.

Then, participants were asked if they are willing to follow the intervention. Those who decided to take part in the intervention were considered the experimental group, and participants who decided not to take part in the intervention were considered the control group. At the start of the intervention, general beverages recommendations were handed out to each participant in the experimental group as a traffic light in which green resembles beverages to drink plenty, orange resembles beverages to drink occasionally, and red resembles beverages to drink rarely, if at all. In addition, each participant was given an individualized daily beverage plan which he/she is recommended to follow for one month providing 10% or less of his/her total energy

Characteristic	n (%)
Gender	
Male	22 (45)
Female	27 (55)
Age	
18 – 25	8 (16)
26 – 35	17 (35)
36 – 49	21 (43)
≥ 50	3 (6)
Medical conditions	
None	43 (88)
Diabetes	4 (8)
Other	2 (4)

TABLE 1: Participants' demographics (n = 49).

needs. Also, participants were provided with a diary in which they were asked to tick the days that they have followed the plan to monitor their progress in the intervention. 10-15 minutes visits were conducted at the end of each week of the intervention for each participant to check his/her diary and to adjust the beverages plan if there is any discomfort.

4. Results

4.1. Participants

Out of 65 residents invited, 49 took part in the study. Table 1 shows the demographic characteristics of 49 residents who were included in the study.

4.2. Beverages Consumption Pattern

Figure 1 shows how often participants drink each type of beverages. The majority (73%) consumed 100% fruit juices with no added sugar. 65% consumed soft drinks, and 60 % consumed plain milk and milk products. Tonic water, energy drinks, sport drinks, and milkshakes are not consumed very often.

Figure 2 shows how often participants drink coffee and tea beverages. The majority (69%) consumed tea beverages rather than coffee beverages. Among all the coffee beverages, American coffee with milk was the most consumed type as 40% drinks

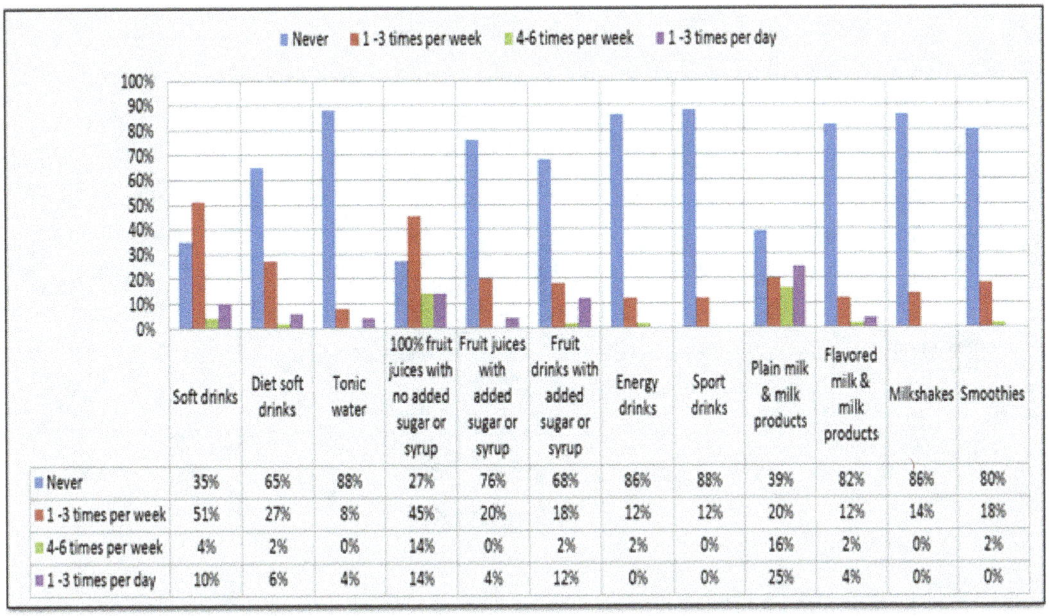

	Soft drinks	Diet soft drinks	Tonic water	100% fruit juices with no added sugar or syrup	Fruit juices with added sugar or syrup	Fruit drinks with added sugar or syrup	Energy drinks	Sport drinks	Plain milk & milk products	Flavored milk & milk products	Milkshakes	Smoothies
Never	35%	65%	88%	27%	76%	68%	86%	88%	39%	82%	86%	80%
1-3 times per week	51%	27%	8%	45%	20%	18%	12%	12%	20%	12%	14%	18%
4-6 times per week	4%	2%	0%	14%	0%	2%	2%	0%	16%	2%	0%	2%
1-3 times per day	10%	6%	4%	14%	4%	12%	0%	0%	25%	4%	0%	0%

Figure 1: Consumption frequency of different types of beverages (n = 49).

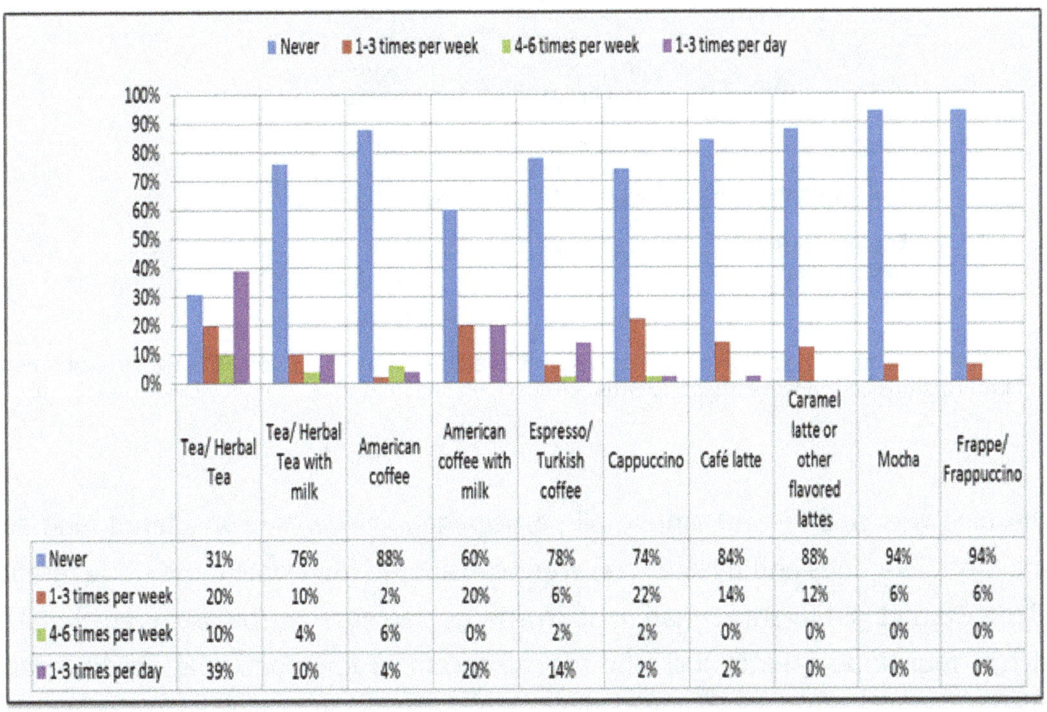

	Tea/ Herbal Tea	Tea/ Herbal Tea with milk	American coffee	American coffee with milk	Espresso/ Turkish coffee	Cappuccino	Café latte	Caramel latte or other flavored lattes	Mocha	Frappe/ Frappuccino
Never	31%	76%	88%	60%	78%	74%	84%	88%	94%	94%
1-3 times per week	20%	10%	2%	20%	6%	22%	14%	12%	6%	6%
4-6 times per week	10%	4%	6%	0%	2%	2%	0%	0%	0%	0%
1-3 times per day	39%	10%	4%	20%	14%	2%	2%	0%	0%	0%

Figure 2: Consumption frequency of coffee and tea beverages (n = 49).

it. Most of the tea and coffee consumers drink their beverage either without sugar or with 1 teaspoon of sugar; it is uncommon for tea and coffee consumers to add 2-3 teaspoons of sugar into their beverage.

55% were overweight or obese, while 45 % had normal weight. Only 29% were within the desirable levels for waist circumference. The mean energy percentage from

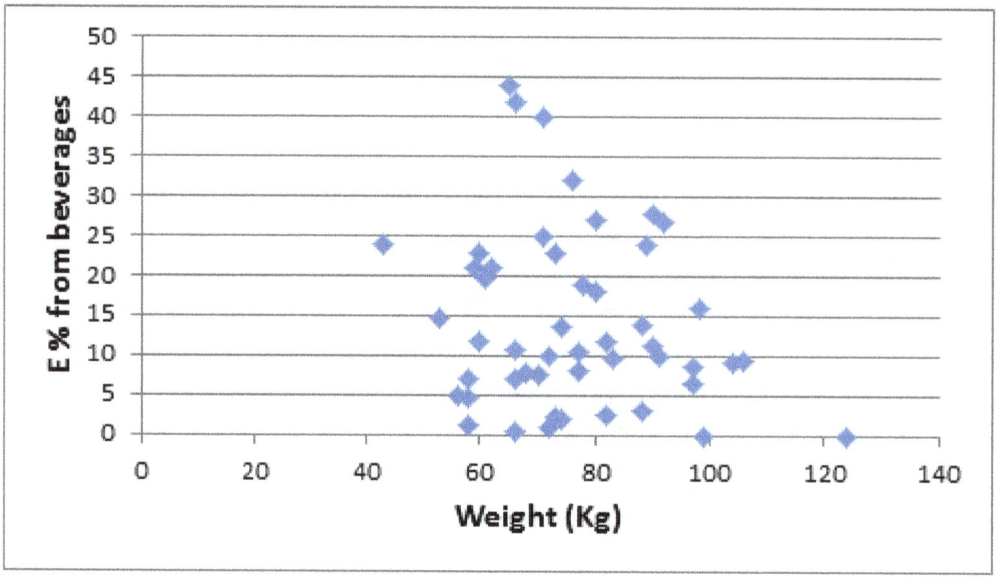

Figure 3: Weight (kg) versus energy percentage from beverages (n = 49).

	Before one-month intervention mean(SD)	After one month intervention mean (SD)	p-value
Weight	78.6 (11.3)	78.2 (11.3)	0.04
Waist Circumference	94.9 (6.7)	94.7 (6.7)	0.08
Energy % from beverages	27.1 (9.6)	12.4 (2.7)	0.0001

TABLE 2: Weight status and energy percentage from beverages of the overweight & obese experimental group before and after one-month intervention.

beverages was 14.2 (± 11.1) among all participants. 53% were considered high consumers of beverages and 47% (n=23) were considered low consumers of beverages. High consumers of beverages had a mean energy percentage from beverages of 22% which is four times greater than the mean percent of low consumers of beverages (5.3%).

Figure 3 shows random, nonlinear relationship between weight and beverages consumption of the 49 participants. This indicates no association between weight & beverages consumption.

Table 2 shows that the one-month intervention was effective in decreasing both the weight and energy percentage of calories from beverages in the overweight & obese experimental group.

5. Discussion

The study found that 37% were overweight and 18% were obese (55% combined). This shows that more than half of the sample falls between overweight and obesity, which reflects the UAE's high rates of overweight, and obesity. Also the results are nearly close to the results of Ng et al. [16] study (with gender differences) that showed that 66.1% of men and 60.6% of women were overweight and obese in 2013.

In addition, our study found that 51% had abdominal obesity, which is associated with a high risk for the diseases including type 2 diabetes, hypertension, dyslipidemia, cardiovascular diseases, and metabolic syndrome. According to the Health Statistics 2012 of Health Authority of Abu Dhabi (2013), the cardiovascular diseases are the first leading cause of deaths in the UAE, and the rates of people who have hypertension and high lipid values are high. Also the UAE is ranked the second highest worldwide for diabetes prevalence. Thus, it can be identified that abdominal obesity is one of the major risks to many health problems in the UAE.

The most frequently consumed beverages (on a daily basis) were plain milk and milk products, 100% fruit juices with no added sugar, and fruit drinks. This reflects that this sample does not consume SSBs on a regular basis and rather they consume them occasionally.

No association was found between weight & beverages consumption. This contradicts with Mozaffarian et al. [15], Basu et al. [1], Tol Chan [4], and Andrew Denmark [6] who all found positive association between SSBs consumption and weight gain. One attributed factor is that this study examined 100% fruit juice and alcohol along with SSBs. According to Tol Chan [4] 100% fruit juices do not associate with BMI, and the present study found that 100% fruit juices is the most consumed beverages which would have affected the results and showed no association. Another attributed factor can be the small sample size. All of the mentioned studies were done on large sample scale, which made it more applicable to identify the association.

Furthermore, the one-month intervention showed that the energy percentage from beverages reduced by 14.7% and the average weight reduced by 0.4 kg in only the overweight & obese participants and not in the normal weight participants. This indicates that the intervention was more effective in reducing energy percentage from beverages and weight for the overweight and obese participants in comparison to normal weight participants.

The reduction in energy percentage from beverages was achievable indicating that overweight and obese participants followed their beverages plan during the one-month period. However, one possible factor that might influence this result is that overweight and obese participants, when they were asked to complete the questionnaire after the intervention, may choose what they were supposed to consume not what they actually consumed. Another factor is that time of the intervention was short which may allow the participant to follow it; however, if it was longer, they may would not manage to follow it.

In addition, the reduction in weight was quick compared to [4] who found that SSBs' reduction was associated with weight loss of 0.49 kg at 6 months and of 0.65 kg at 18 months. This indicates that possibly other factors have impacted the results. One factor is that overweight and obese participants may have a heavy meal when they were measured before the intervention, which they may did not have when they were measured after the intervention. Other factor is that maybe overweight and obese participants were encouraged to lose weight when they were told about the intervention, so they did other lifestyle/diet modifications besides beverages' reduction.

6. Limitations

Limitations of this study include the limited time of the intervention (only one month), as well as the small sample size that was not a representative sample for Al Reef residential compound. In addition, this study studied the combined effect of SSBs, 100% fruit juices, and alcohol consumption on weight status and did not examined the separated effect of each type of beverages. Furthermore, this study focused on beverages consumption in relation to weight status and did not take into account other dietary factors that impact weight status including food and eating habits.

7. Conclusion

The study highlighted major health problems in Abu Dhabi including high rates of overweight, obesity, and abdominal obesity. Plain milk and milk products, fruit juices, and fruit drinks were the most frequently consumed beverages and tea seemed more popular than coffee. The one-month intervention was effective in reducing the energy percentage from beverages and weight of the overweight and obese participants, but no association was found in this sample between beverages consumption and overweight and obesity. Further studies on larger scale of participants and time are needed to investigate the association between beverages consumption and overweight and obesity, and to examine the effectiveness of reducing beverages consumption on weight loss.

8. Acknowledgements

The researcher thanks the following individuals for their support of this research:

Residents from Al Reef Villas (Abu Dhabi), for their participation in the study and in the intervention for nothing just for their health welfare.

Dr. Malin Garemo, study supervisor, for her comprehensive and professional support and advice and for her continuous encouragement throughout the study.

My family for their continuous encouragement and emotional support throughout the study.

References

[1] S. Basu, M. McKee, G. Galea, and D. Stuckler, "Relationship of soft drink consumption to global overweight, obesity, and diabetes: A cross-national analysis of 75 countries," *American Journal of Public Health*, vol. 103, no. 11, pp. 2071–2077, 2013.

[2] L. A. Bazzano, T. Y. Li, K. J. Joshipura, and F. B. Hu, "Intake of fruit, vegetables, and fruit juices and risk of diabetes in women," *Diabetes Care*, vol. 31, no. 7, pp. 1311–1317, 2008.

[3] B. A. Burt, J. L. Kolker, A. M. Sandretto, Y. Yuan, W. Sohn, and A. I. Ismail, "Dietary patterns related to caries in a low-income adult population," *Caries Research*, vol. 40, no. 6, pp. 473–480, 2006.

[4] T. Chan, "Sugar-Sweetened Beverage Consumption Frequency vs," in *BMI, National Health and Nutrition Examination Survey 2003-2004.Thesis*, Georgia State University, 2011.

[5] L. Chen, L. J. Appel, C. Loria et al., "Reduction in consumption of sugar-sweetened beverages is associated with weight loss: The PREMIER trial," *American Journal of Clinical Nutrition*, vol. 89, no. 5, pp. 1299–1306, 2009.

[6] A. Denmark, *The Effect of SSB Intake on BMI of College Students at the University of Kentucky*, University of Kentucky, 2012.

[7] P. Fellows and A. Hampton, Small-scale food processing - A guide for appropriate equipment. London: Intermediate Technology Publications 1992.

[8] L. Harnack, J. Stang, and M. Story, "Soft drink consumption among US children and adolescents: Nutritional consequences," *Journal of the Academy of Nutrition and Dietetics*, vol. 99, no. 4, pp. 436–441, 1999.

[9] *Health Authority Abu Dhabi*, Health Statistics, 2012.

[10] M. Inoue-Choi, K. Robien, A. Mariani, J. R. Cerhan, and K. E. Anderson, "Sugar-sweetened beverage intake and the risk of type I and type II endometrial cancer

among postmenopausal women," *Cancer Epidemiology, Biomarkers & Prevention*, vol. 22, no. 12, pp. 2384–2394, 2013.

[11] B. W. Jensen, M. Nichols, S. Allender et al., "Inconsistent associations between sweet drink intake and 2-year change in BMI among Victorian children and adolescents," *Pediatric Obesity*, vol. 8, no. 4, pp. 271–283, 2013.

[12] B. K. Kit, T. H. I. Fakhouri, S. Park, S. J. Nielsen, and C. L. Ogden, "Trends in sugar-sweetened beverage consumption among youth and adults in the United States: 1999-2010," *American Journal of Clinical Nutrition*, vol. 98, no. 1, pp. 180–188, 2013.

[13] J. L. Kolker, Y. Yuan, B. A. Burt et al., "Dental caries and dietary patterns in low-income African American children," *Journal of Pediatric Dentistry*, vol. 29, no. 6, pp. 457–464, 2007.

[14] V. S. Malik, B. M. Popkin, G. A. Bray, J.-P. Després, W. C. Willett, and F. B. Hu, "Sugar-sweetened beverages and risk of metabolic syndrome and type 2 diabetes: a meta-analysis," *Diabetes Care*, vol. 33, no. 11, pp. 2477–2483, 2010.

[15] D. Mozaffarian, T. Hao, E. B. Rimm, W. C. Willett, and F. B. Hu, "Changes in diet and lifestyle and long-term weight gain in women and men," *The New England Journal of Medicine*, vol. 364, no. 25, pp. 2392–2404, 2011.

[16] M. Ng, T. Fleming, M. Robinson et al., "Global, regional, and national prevalence of overweight and obesity in children and adults during 1980–2013: a systematic analysis for the Global Burden of Disease Study 2013," *The Lancet*, vol. 384, no. 9945, pp. 766–781, 2014.

[17] B. M. Popkin, L. E. Armstrong, G. M. Bray, B. Caballero, B. Frei, and W. C. Willett, "A new proposed guidance system for beverage consumption in the United States," *American Journal of Clinical Nutrition*, vol. 83, no. 3, pp. 529–542, 2006.

[18] F. Rodríguez-Artalejo, E. López García, L. Gorgojo et al., "Consumption of bakery products, sweetened soft drinks and yogurt among children aged 6-7 years: Association with nutrient intake and overall diet quality," *British Journal of Nutrition*, vol. 89, no. 3, pp. 419–428, 2003.

[19] Wood. Robert, *Johnson Foundation. The Negative Impact of Sugar-Sweetened Beverages on Childrens Health*, University of Minnesota, School of Public Health, 2009.

[20] The CDC Guide to Strategies for Reducing the Consumption of Sugar-Sweetened Beverages, 2010.

[21] The Department of Nutrition at Harvard School of Public Health, FACT SHEET: Sugary drink supersizing and the obesity epidemic. 2012.

[22] J. J. Warren, K. Weber-Gasparoni, T. A. Marshall et al., "A longitudinal study of dental caries risk among very young low SES children," *Community Dentistry and Oral Epidemiology*, vol. 37, no. 2, pp. 116–122, 2009.

[23] S. W. Ng, C. Ni Mhurchu, S. A. Jebb, and B. M. Popkin, "Patterns and trends of beverage consumption among children and adults in Great Britain, 1986–2009," *British Journal of Nutrition*, vol. 108, no. 3, pp. 536–551, 2012.

[24] S. W. Ng, S. Zaghloul, H. Ali et al., "Nutrition transition in the United Arab Emirates," *European Journal of Clinical Nutrition*, vol. 65, no. 12, pp. 1328–1337, 2011.

18

Educator's ability to identify students with coordination disorders

Michalis Anastasiadis[1], Thomas Kourtessis[2], and Evridiki Zachopoulou[3]

[1]Department of Life & Health Sciences, University of Nicosia, 46, Makedonitissas Avenue, Nicosia, Cyprus
[2]Department of Physical Education & Sport Science, Democritus University of Thrace, University Campus, Komotini, Greece
[3]Department of Early Childhood Care and Education, Alexander Technological Educational Institute of Thessaloniki, Greece

Corresponding Author: Michalis Anastasiadis; email: anastasiades.m@cytanet.com.cy

Abstract

According to research 5-7% of the total school population face motor learning difficulties such as Developmental Coordination Disorder (DCD). In addition to that, recent findings regarding comorbidity revealed that specific learning difficulties such as Dyslexia are very often co-exist with movement difficulties such as DCD. School environment seems to be an ideal setting for early identification, assessment and in-school intervention. Therefore, educators' knowledge regarding DCD and their ability to identify and assess children with movement difficulties are crucial dimensions for an effective interventional management. The goal of the current paper was a review of the relative literature. The findings reveal that, without specific education, the educators have limited ability to recognize children with DCD. Furthermore, research has shown that well informed and educated educators can be very effective in identification and classification of students with movement difficulties. As a result, early intervention strategies can be developed and applied to help the students and their families. Therefore the current article provides a review of literature regarding the ability of the educators to identify their students with motor coordination difficulties. A review of the most commonly used identification instruments was also provided.

Keywords: Developmental Coordination Disorder, identification, assessment

1. Introduction

Developmental Coordination Disorder (DCD) has been recognized as one of the six most common developmental disorders in childhood [27, 39] and refers to motor performance that is substantially below expected levels, given the person's chronologic age, which significantly interferes with activities of daily living during childhood, and is not due to a known general medical condition [1, 2]. In addition to that "Developmental coordination disorder is diagnosed only if the impairment in motor skills significantly interferes with the performance of, or participation in, daily activities in family, social, school, or community life. Examples of such activities include using specific tools in class such as rulers and scissors, and participating in team exercise activities at school. Not only is ability to perform these actions impaired, but also marked slowness in execution is common. Handwriting competence is frequently affected, consequently affecting legibility and/or speed of written output and affecting academic achievement" [1].

Research has revealed that children with DCD have below average physical conditions [5, 13, 32], are not physically active [6, 42], and are at high risk of obesity levels that leads to type-II diabetes [4, 13, 16]. Apart from the motor domain, these children may experience social and emotional deficiencies [7], low self-esteem, isolation from friends, and reduced participation in games [28, 34]. Children with DCD find it difficult to compete in strength, speed and skill in games with their peers as they make comparisons that result in personal failure and thus lower self-esteem. Finally, a growing body of literature regarding comorbidity suggests that deficits in motor skill performance frequently exist among children with learning disabilities [21], such as dyslexia [37] and Attention Deficit Hyperactivity Disorder [25].

The importance of early motor identification and assessment has been early highlighted (Miyahara, Kaplan, Crawford & Wilson, 2002; Larkin & Rose, 2005). However, it seems rather impossible for all preschoolers and early school-aged students to be assessed. Therefore, it seems crucial for educators to be able to screen and identify students with motor coordination difficulties [12]. The school environment seems the ideal environment for early detection of children with DCD. In schools the teachers spend many hours with children daily, that are familiar with the schools 'friendly and pleasant environment. Early and accurate identification and assessment leads to individualized and effective intervention strategies. The current article provides a review of literature regarding the ability of the educators to identify their students with motor coordination difficulties. A review of the most commonly used identification instruments was also provided.

2. Methods

The search for available articles on educator's ability to identify students with DCD was made through the widely used databases PubMed, ERIC, Medline, EBSCO, Scopus, SportDiscus. There was no chronological limitation to the search, other than that defined by the database itself. The keywords introduced were Developmental Coordination Disorder, identification, motor assessment, only studies related to the teacher's ability to recognize students with developmental coordination disorders were selected.

3. Educators' ability to identify movement difficulties

The knowledge of the teachers for the first identification of children with motor disorders is very important but even more vital is the ability of systematic intervention for effective and faster intervention. Two studies investigated the specific knowledge regarding Developmental Coordination Disorder among classroom teachers and physical educators in Greece and Cyprus [3, 38]. Both studies confirmed the limited knowledge of the educators in regard to Development Disorders and Movement Coordination. In addition, further data analysis revealed that there was no significant correlation between years of previous work experience and specific knowledge [3]. Participants of both studies expressed their belief that they would benefit from specific ongoing education and training.

In their study on 70 ten year-old boys, Morris and Winter (1971), found that teachers were able to recognize correctly 50% of children had movement disorders. In another study, Keogh, Sugden, Raynald, & Calkins (1979) stated that teachers who participated in the investigation could not identify more than 20%-30% of cases of children with physical clumsiness. Accordingly, Revie and Larkin (1993) declared that teachers who participated in their research, showed low recognition capability (42%), when they evaluated children in the age range 5-9. Similarly, Sovik and Maeland (1986) found that the teachers identified eight out of the 21 children to have motor/ kinetic difficulties, while seven children with motor disorders were not recognized.

Wilson, Neil, Kamps, and Babcock, (2012) studied the awareness of family doctors, pediatricians, school teachers and parents to identify movement disorders in children. The findings suggested that compared to other mental disorders, they also were not able to identify motor disorders such as, motor learning disability, dyspraxia, developmental coordination disorder and clumsy child syndrome.

It is important that teachers receive more training regarding movement difficulties and how they affect children. The school is often the primary source of reference, as the teachers are the first to observe poor developmental children's skills to interfere with classroom work and overall academic performance [36]. While secondary school teachers have shown that they are more capable to identify some children with DCD, the literature suggests that primary teachers cannot distinguish those children and this may be related to various factors such as the lack of knowledge [11, 15, 19, 29]. One solution to these problems is the control and observation checklists on motor disorders to be distributed to the teachers, but apparently do not work well, as they are often extensive and time consuming [17]. Piek and Edwards (1997) evaluated the ability of teachers and physical education teachers to identify children with motor coordination problems using the Movement Assessment Battery for Children (MABC; Henderson & Sugden, 1994). The results showed that the teachers were able to identify 25% of children with DCD, and physical education teachers were able to identify 49%. However, this was expected due to the nature of the profession. Physical education teachers are responsible for physical education, so they have a better ability to observe the mobility of children. The fact that in countries like Cyprus the lesson of physical education is taught by elementary school teachers results in the lack of teaching basic skills to children of these ages, as well as the lack of teachers' experiences of perceiving children's motor weaknesses. In South Africa, physical education was rejected by South African schools as an autonomous topic and they still do not receive a targeted physical education program at school [8].

The teachers have excellent opportunities to observe children in their daily lives in various movement activities in the classroom [24]. Nevertheless, according to Gubbay (1975) it seems that the teachers have low ability to identify the DCD. In alignment with this statement other researchers [9, 12, 22] agreed that most teachers do not have the knowledge to identify children with motor disorders. Ellinoudis and colleagues (2009) explored the ability of Physical Educators to identify movement difficulties among 340 primary education children. According to the results educators exhibited a low identification ability recognizing correctly only 27% of the 59 children with severe and moderate movement difficulties. On the other hand, they were able to identify with relative accuracy all the children without any motor difficulties, thus revealing a lack of specific knowledge regarding this issue. The important role of specific training of educators regarding identification of students with movement difficulties has been shown by Kourtessis and colleagues (2009). The purpose of this study was to investigate whether an educational program focused on specific issues regarding motor learning disorders would enhance the educators' ability to recognize and identify students with such difficulties. Both kindergarten and physical education teachers were randomly assigned into an experimental and a control group. Participants of the control group were asked to identify children with motor difficulties without any previous information whereas their colleagues of the experimental group were asked to do the same after a 3-week intensive educational program. The results revealed that whereas the educators of the control group exhibited low identification ability, their trained participants showed significantly higher identification ability. Furthermore, an interesting finding was that non-trained kindergarten teachers exhibited higher identification ability compared to their non-trained physical education colleagues. The researchers concluded that the specific training had a positive effect on the educators' ability to identify children with movement difficulties. Therefore, continuing education on similar issues should be an integral part of any educational system.

The studies mentioned above, focused on the ability of teachers to identify motor disorders. The following table summarizes the various studies, the instruments they were used and the results. Most of the studies imply that primary school teachers have limited familiarity and knowledge to identify children with motor disorders. Yet, this identification seems to be easier for physical education teachers but still have their own weaknesses.

4. Checklists and Questionnaires for teachers

An equally important part are the questionnaires and checklists used by teachers to be able to detect children with mobility difficulties. Listed below are the most popular instruments of this kind (Table 2).

The Movement Assessment Battery for Children 2 Checklist [19] which has been designed to serve as a first screening in the identification process. This is done based on a list of specific motor behaviors that can be observed in an everyday setting such as a classroom or playground. A child's performance on each item is rated by an adult observer in terms of how competently it is executed. These ratings are summed to provide a total score, which is then mapped onto a 'Traffic Light' system showing whether a child falls into the age-appropriate range (green zone), shows some delay or some minor movement problems that need to be monitored (amber zone) or is highly likely to have a more severe movement problem (red zone). The checklist has been designed to be used by Physical Education teachers, classroom teachers, parents, therapists and other professionals involved with children who have movement difficulties [19]. The

Authors	Instruments	Results	Weaknesses
Gubbay 1975	Questionnaire	Teachers have low ability to identify the DCD. It was much lower than 50%.	- Teachers recognized more girls than boys, something that does not agree most of research.
Ellinoudis et al 2009	Movement ABC-Checklist	Teachers have low ability to identify the DCD. (27.1%)	The age of children was a factor that may affected physical education teachers, since they failed to successfully recognize children of the 6th grade
Kourtessis et al 2008	Movement ABC-Checklist	Teachers have low ability to identify the DCD	Relatively small sample
Sovik & Maeland 1986	-Test of Motor Proficiency -Test of motor impairment -Questionnaire	-Teachers' ratings of clumsiness had low correlation with criteria of clumsiness derived from the performance tests -The teachers identified 8 out of the 21 children to have motor/ kinetic difficulties, while 7 children with motor disorders were not recognized.	-Only children aged 9 years. -Although no systematic examination could be done in regard to articulation, social and emotional problems among subjects within the sample of clumsy children, some information of this kind was collected from their teachers. -The two tests and the questionnaire detect different children: TOMI 52% TMP 39%
Revie & Larkin, 1993	BMAT-R Checklist	Teachers have low recognition capability (42%),	- Small sample. - Only the gross motor of children was evaluated.
Junaid et al 2000	Movement ABC-Checklist	Teachers cannot identify children with motor coordination problems. - They recognized only children (3.9%) with severe motor problems.	- The teachers criticized the checklist for being too long and time consuming to complete. - The 32 participating educators were not taught how to complete the checklist. They were just given the few instructions that were included in the test kit. -Language expression and understanding may have affected the exposure of children to certain tests on the checklist and influenced the teachers and graded them graciously on the checklist.

TABLE 1: Summary of the main studies on teachers' familiarity to identify motor disorders.

Authors	Instruments	Results	Weaknesses
Piek & Edwards 1997	Movement ABC-Checklist [18]	Teachers could identify 25% of children with DCD but the physical education teachers were able to identify 49% of DCD children.	Lack of experience of Classroom teachers regarding the movement characteristics of the children
Milander 2016	Movement Assessment Battery for Children – Test & Checklist	The ability of teachers to use the MABC-C to correctly identify children with motor difficulties was low.	- An important factor that may have influenced teachers' low knowledge is that in South African schools they do not teach physical education lessons that result in children's poor motor skills. - In addition, Kinder kineticists and teachers have different backgrounds and experiences and may have influenced the outcome. Some of the teachers have several years of experience in motor development

Table 1: Table Continued.

MABC-2 Checklist was used in the present project as an identification criterion to be decided if a case demanded further motor assessment.

The Developmental Disorder Coordination Questionnaire'07 [41] is a questionnaire for parents and teachers of 5 to 15 year old children and includes 15 questions rated on a 5 point-scale (1=not at all like your child; 5=extremely like your child). The total score ranged from 15 to 75. A lower score indicates suspicion of DCD. Different cutoff scores were established for different categories of ages. Below 8 years, the cutoff is ≤46, for children between 8 and 10 years, the cutoff is ≤55 and for children above 10 years, the cutoff is ≤57. The items are classified in three factors (1) control during movement, (2) fine motor/handwriting, and (3) general coordination.

The Motor Observation Questionnaire - T (MOQ-T) is a questionnaire for teachers and is aimed at children aged 5 to 11 years. This questionnaire was developed in the Netherlands and its previous version was the Groningen Motor Observation Scale (van Dellen & Kalverboer, 1987) which was aimed at children aged 6-11 years and was then extended to include children aged 5 years. The MOQ-T was adapted based on reliability data that used a large database of 1919 children to compose the new rules [34]. The

Checklists and questionnaires	Year	Age	Objectives
Movement Assessment Battery for Children 2 Checklist	Henderson , Sugden & Barnett, 2007	From 5 to 12 years old	A list of specific motor behaviours that can be observed in an everyday setting. Focuses on how a child manages daily tasks at home and at school.
Developmental Disorder Coordination Questionnaire'07	Wilson, Kaplan, Crawford & Roberts, 2007	From 5 to 15 years old	Control during movement. Fine motor/handwriting. General coordination.
Motor Observation Questionnaire - T (MOQ-T)	Previous version was the Groningen Motor Observation Scale (van Dellen & Kalverboer, 1987) Schoemaker, 2003	Children aged 5 to 11 years	Fine and gross motor functioning. Identify children with DCD or clumsiness.
Children Activity Scales for Teachers (ChAS-T)	Rosenblum, 2006	Children aged 4-8	Activities of daily living (ADLs) skills. Organization in time and space. Motor performance

TABLE 2: The most popular questionnaires and checklists.

original questionnaire included 20 items and then adjusted to 18 items rated on a 4-point scale (1 = never valid, 4 = always valid) with the total score ranging from 18-72. The high score of the questionnaire shows that the child is at risk of DCD.

The Children Activity Scales for Teachers (ChAS-T) is a questionnaire developed in Israel and can be used by teachers in children aged 4-8 who are at risk for DCD [32]. It contains 21 items that are similar to Children Activity Scales for Parents (ChAS-P). Due to the fact that teachers were having difficulty with some questions, 6 elements from the daily living activity of ChAS-P were removed. ChAS-T has been developed to provide information on how children work in everyday life in the natural environment. These elements relate to organizing space and time in day-to-day activities, gambling activities, ball skills, mobility, joint school and preschool activities and academic ability. Its credibility and validity regarding the ChAS-T scale has been examined with encouraging results [32].

5. Conclusion

According to De Milander and colleagues (2016) the ability of teachers to recognize children with DCD is rather low and perhaps an important factor may be their limited knowledge regarding coordination disorders. If the teachers are not properly educated and especially trained during their basic studies, they cannot identify and properly evaluate these children. On the contrary, well trained and educated teachers can have a very good effect to identify and correctly classify children with mobility disabilities [22]. The importance of early assessment and diagnosis of children with disabilities has been stressed repeatedly by most researchers. Yet, it is practically impossible to assess all students of primary schools of a country. Hence, teachers and especially physical education teachers could play a key role in identifying these children and, then, refer the children for further evaluation to experts (Kourtessis, 1997). In the last decades, teachers emphasize on the agility of movement, in order to teach other fields as mathematics, geography, etc. Thus, the importance of proper and timely identification of children with difficulties in movement in order to receive the necessary assistance, is evident [22].

In conclusion, as we have seen in the above review, teachers' ability to correctly identify children with developmental coordination disorders is moderate to low. Although the literature shows that physical education teachers are more capable than primary school teachers in identifying children with DCD, they still do not have the sufficient ability to recognize all of these children. Trained and educated teachers can be very effective in identifying and classifying children with movement difficulties. Motor assessment combined with the Questionnaires/Checklist are a very good evaluation tool for children with movement disorders. Therefore, it is very important for teachers to use the Questionnaires / Checklists on children who have indications that they may present DCD. Professional training and relevant future research for teacher education appear to be justified and necessary.

References

[1] American Psychiatric Association. (2013). Diagnostic and Statistical Manual of Mental Disorders (5th ed.). Washington, DC: Authors

[2] American Psychiatric Association. (1994). Diagnostic and Statistical Manual of Mental Disorders (4th ed.). Washington, DC: Authors

[3] Anastasiadis, M., Kourtessis, T., Zisi, V. & Kioumourtzoglou, E. (2016). Knowledge of elementary school educators in Cyprus regarding developmental coordination disorder in childhood. Journal of Physical Activity, Nutrition and Rehabilitation, August 12, http://www.panr.com.cy/?p=1495.

[4] Cairney, J., Hay J.A., Faught, B.E., Hawes, R. (2005). Developmental coordination disorder and overweight and obesity in children aged 9-14 years. International Journal of Obesity, 29, 369-372.

[5] Cairney, J., Hay J.A., Faught, B.E., Flouris, A., Klentrou, P. (2007). Developmental coordination disorder and cardiorespiratory fitness in children. Paediatric Exercise Science, 19, 20-28.

[6] Cairney, J., Kwan, M. Y. W., Hay, J., & Faught, B. E. (2012). Developmental coordination disorder, gender and body weight: Examining the impact of participation in active play. Research in Developmental Disabilities, 33, 1566-1573.

[7] Candell, M. H., Smyth, M. M. & Ahonen, T. P. (1994) Clumsiness in adolescence: Educational, motor and social outcomes of motor delay detected at 5 years. Adapted Physical Activity Quarterly, 11, 115-129.

[8] Cleophas, F.J. (2014). A historical-political perspective on Physical Education in South Africa during the period 1990-1999. South African Journal for Research in Sport, Physical Education and Recreation, 36(1), 11-27.

[9] De Milander, M., Coetzee, F.F., Venter, A. (2016). Prevalence and effect of developmental coordination disorder on learning-related skills of South African grade one children. South African Journal for Research in Sport, Physical Education and Recreation. 38(2), 49-62

[10] Dewey, D., Kaplan, B.J., Crawford, S.G., & Wilson, B.N. (2002). Developmental coordination disorder: Associated problems in attention, learning and psychosocial adjustment. Human Movement Science, 21, 905-918.

[11] Dunford, C., Street, E., O'Connell, H., Kelly, J., & Sibert, J. R. (2004). Are referrals to occupational therapy for developmental coordination disorder appropriate? Archives of Disease in Childhood, 89(2), 143-147.

[12] Ellinoudis, T., Kiparissis, M. Gitsas, K. & Kourtessis, T. (2009). Ability to detect movement difficulties in children aged 7-12 years by physical education teachers using the assessment package Movement Assessment Battery for Children. Physical Education & Sports, 29(3), 288-306.

[13] Faught, B.E., Hay, J.A., Cairney, J., Flouris A. (2005). Increased risk for coronary vascular disease in children with developmental coordination disorder. Journal of Adolescent Health, 37, 376-80.

[14] Gubbay, S.S. (1975). Clumsy children in normal schools. The Medical Journal of Australia, 1, 233-236

[15] Green, D., Bishop, T., Wilson, B., Crawford, S., Hooper, R., Kaplan, B., et al. (2005). Is questionnaire-based screening part of the solution to waiting lists for children with, developmental coordination disorder? British Journal of Occupational Therapy, 68, 2-10

[16] Hay, J. A., Hawes, R., & Faught, B. E. (2004). Evaluation of a screening instrument for developmental coordination disorder. Journal of Adolescent Health: Official Publication of the Society for Adolescent Medicine, 34, 308-313.

[17] Henderson, S.E., Sugden, D.A. (1992). Movement Assessment Battery for Children: Manual. London: Psychological Corporation.

[18] Henderson, S.E., Sugden, D.A., & Barnett, A.L. (2007). Movement Assessment Battery for Children - 2. Examiner's Manual. U.K.: Harcourt Assessment

[19] Junaid, K., Harris, S.R., Fulmer, A., & Carswell, A. (2000). Teachers' use of the MABC Checklist to identify children with motor difficulties. Pediatric Physical Therapy, 12, 158-163

[20] Keogh, J.F., Sugden, D.A. Raynald, C.L. & Calkins, J.A. (1979). Identification of clumsy children: Comparisons and comments. Journal of Human Movement Studies, 5, 32-41.

[21] Kourtessis T., Thomaidou E., Liveri-Kantere A., Michalopoulou M., Kourtessis A., & Kioumourtzoglou E. (2008). Prevalence of developmental coordination disorder among Greek children with learning disabilities-A preliminary study. European Psychomotricity Journal, 1(2), 10-17.

[22] Kourtessis, T., Tzetzis, G., Kioumourtzoglou, E., & Mavromatis, G. (2001). The effects of an intensive recreational intervention program on children with movement difficulties. New Zealand Journal of Disability Studies, 9, 120-139.

[23] Kourtessis, T., Tsigilis, N., Maheridou, M., Ellinoudis, T., Kiparissis, M. & Kioumourtzoglou, E. (2008). The Influence of a short intervention program on early childhood and physical education teacher ability to identify children with developmental coordination disorders. Journal of Early Childhood Teacher Education, 2(4), 276-286

[24] Larkin, D., & Rose, E. (2005). Assessment of developmental coordination disorder. In D. A. Sugden & M. E.Chambers (Eds.), Children with developmental coordination disorder (pp. 135-154). London: Whurr Publishers Ltd.

[25] Miyahara, M., Mobs, I. & Doll-Tepper, G. (2001). Severity of hyperactivity and the comorbidity of hyperactivity with clumsiness in three sample sources: school, support group and hospital. Child: Care, Health and Development, 27, 5, 413-424.

[26] Morris, R. & Winter, M. (1971). Identifying clumsy children: Validation of the Stott test of motor impairment in the school situation. Journal of Human Movement Studies, 4, 4-8.

[27] Orton, S.T. (1937). Reading, writing, and speech problems in children. New York: Norton.

[28] Piek, J.B., Bayman, G.B. & Barnett. N.C. (2006). The relationship between fine and gross motor ability, self-perception and self-wort in children and adolescents. Human Movement Science, 25(11), 65-75.

[29] Piek, J.P., & Edwards, K. (1997). The identification of children with developmental coordination disorder by class and physical education teachers. British Journal of Educational Psychology, 67, 55-67.

[30] Revie, G., Larkin, D. (1993). Task specific intervention with children reduces movement problems. Adapted Physical Activities Quarterly, 4, 29-41.

[31] Rosenblum S (2006). The development and standardization of the Children Activity Scales (ChAS-P/T) for the early identification of children with Developmental Coordination Disorders. Child Care & Health Development, 32, 619-632.

[32] Schott, N., Alof, V., Hultsch, D., & Meermann, D. (2007). Physical fitness in children with developmental coordination disorder. Research Quarterly for Exercise & Sport, 78, 438-50

[33] Schoemaker, M. M. (2003). Manual of the motor observation questionnaire for teachers. Groningen: Internal Publication, Center for Human Movement Sciences, In Dutch.

[34] Skinner, R.A., Piek, J.P. (2001). Psychosocial implications of poor motor coordination in children and adolescents. Human Movement Science, 20, 73-94.

[35] Sovik, N., & Maeland, A.F. (1986). Children with motor problems (clumsy children). Scandinavian Journal of Educational Research, 30(1), 39-53.

[36] Sugden, D. A. & Wright H. C. (1998). Motor coordination disorders in children. California: Sage publications.

[37] Tziva-Kostala, V., Kourtessis, T., Kostala, M., Michalopoulou, M. & Evaggelinou, C. (2011). Coordination Disorder in Children with Dyslexia. European Psychomotricity Journal, 4(1), 29-37.

[38] Tziva-Kostala, V., Douroukas, K., Kostala, A., & Kourtessis, T. (2008). Pilot recording of Teacher Knowledge for Developmental Co-ordination Disorder. Proceedings of the National Congress in Health-Environment-Education: Questions & Suggestions (pp. 77-83). National & Kapodistrian University of Athens, Department of Biology. Athens, 27-28 March 2009.

[39] Wall, A.E., Reid, G., & Paton, J. (1990). The syndrome of physical awkwardness. In G. Reid (Ed.), Problems in movement control. North-Holland: Elsevier Science Publishers B.V.

[40] Wilson, B.N., Kaplan, B.J., Crawford, S.G. & Roberts, G. (2007). The developmental coordination disorder questionnaire (DCDQ). Available: http://www.dcdq.ca/

[41] Wilson, B. N., Neil, K., Kamps, P. H. and Babcock, S. (2012). Awareness and knowledge of developmental co-ordination disorder among physicians, teachers and

[42] Wrotniak, B. H., Epstein, L. H., Dorn, J. M., Jones, K. E., & Kondilis, V. A. (2006). The relationship between motor proficiency and physical activity in children. Paediatrics, 118, e1758-e1765.

PERMISSIONS

All chapters in this book were first published in AJNE, by Knowledge E; hereby published with permission under the Creative Commons Attribution License or equivalent. Every chapter published in this book has been scrutinized by our experts. Their significance has been extensively debated. The topics covered herein carry significant findings which will fuel the growth of the discipline. They may even be implemented as practical applications or may be referred to as a beginning point for another development.

The contributors of this book come from diverse backgrounds, making this book a truly international effort. This book will bring forth new frontiers with its revolutionizing research information and detailed analysis of the nascent developments around the world.

We would like to thank all the contributing authors for lending their expertise to make the book truly unique. They have played a crucial role in the development of this book. Without their invaluable contributions this book wouldn't have been possible. They have made vital efforts to compile up to date information on the varied aspects of this subject to make this book a valuable addition to the collection of many professionals and students.

This book was conceptualized with the vision of imparting up-to-date information and advanced data in this field. To ensure the same, a matchless editorial board was set up. Every individual on the board went through rigorous rounds of assessment to prove their worth. After which they invested a large part of their time researching and compiling the most relevant data for our readers.

The editorial board has been involved in producing this book since its inception. They have spent rigorous hours researching and exploring the diverse topics which have resulted in the successful publishing of this book. They have passed on their knowledge of decades through this book. To expedite this challenging task, the publisher supported the team at every step. A small team of assistant editors was also appointed to further simplify the editing procedure and attain best results for the readers.

Apart from the editorial board, the designing team has also invested a significant amount of their time in understanding the subject and creating the most relevant covers. They scrutinized every image to scout for the most suitable representation of the subject and create an appropriate cover for the book.

The publishing team has been an ardent support to the editorial, designing and production team. Their endless efforts to recruit the best for this project, has resulted in the accomplishment of this book. They are a veteran in the field of academics and their pool of knowledge is as vast as their experience in printing. Their expertise and guidance has proved useful at every step. Their uncompromising quality standards have made this book an exceptional effort. Their encouragement from time to time has been an inspiration for everyone.

The publisher and the editorial board hope that this book will prove to be a valuable piece of knowledge for researchers, students, practitioners and scholars across the globe.

LIST OF CONTRIBUTORS

Galanis Nikiforos, Alafropatis Ilias, Tsiridis Eleftherios, Sayegh Fares and Kirkos John
Division of Sports Medicine, Department of Orthopaedics, Papageorgiou General Hospital, Medical School, Aristotle University of Thessaloniki, Greece

Kleftouris George
Royal Lancaster Infirmary University Hospital, NHS trust, Lancaster, UK

Oral Onur
School of Physical Education and Sports, Ege University, Izmir, Turkey

Shaimaa S. Altunaiji, Mariam Muayyad and Zainab Ali
Department of Clinical Nutrition and Dietetics, College of Health Sciences, University of Sharjah, Sharjah, UAE

Amita Attlee, Mona Hashim and Reyad S. Obaid
Department of Clinical Nutrition and Dietetics, College of Health Sciences, University of Sharjah, Sharjah, UAE
Research Institute of Medical and Health Sciences, University of Sharjah, Sharjah, UAE

Chara Odysseos and Maria Avraamidou
Department of Life and Health Sciences, University of Nicosia, Cyprus

Teresa Arora
Zayed University, Department of Psychology, Abu Dhabi, United Arab Emirates
Weill Cornell Medicine in Qatar, Clinical Research Core, Doha, Qatar

Sahar Agouba Ahmad Sharara and Shahrad Taheri
Weill Cornell Medicine in Qatar, Clinical Research Core, Doha, Qatar

Sousana Papadopoulou, Elpiniki Kroustalloudi, Anna Kokkinopoulou and Maria Hassapidou
Department of Nutrition & Dietetics, Alexander Technological Educational Institute of Thessaloniki, Sindos, Thessaloniki, Greece

Ioannis Pagkalos
Department of Nutrition & Dietetics, Alexander Technological Educational Institute of Thessaloniki, Sindos, Thessaloniki, Greece
Department of Electrical & Computer Engineering, Aristotle University of Thessaloniki, Thessaloniki, Greece

Zainab Taha and Ayesha S. Rashed
College of Narural and Health Sciences, Zayed University, Abu Dhabi, U.A.E

Dimitrios Papandreou
Department of Health Sciences, Zayed University, Abu Dhabi, United Arab Emirates

Al-Nasraween M
Food and Drug Administration, Food Control Department, Amman, Jordan

Al Omari L, Al-Jaghbeer M and Al-Qutob R
Community Health Department, Faculty of Medicine, University of Jordan, Amman, Jordan

Berggren V
Faculty of Health Sciences, Lund University, Lund, Sweden
Department of Neuroscience, caring science and society, Karolinska Institutet, Stockholm, Sweden

Taha H
Community Health Department, Faculty of Medicine, University of Jordan, Amman, Jordan
Faculty of Health Sciences, Lund University, Lund, Sweden

Elham A. Aljaaly
King Abdul-Aziz University, Saudi Arabia

Eiman Al Hammadi
Department of Natural Sciences and Public Health, Zayed University, Abudhabi, UAE

Marcou Juliana and Savva Rafaella-Maria
Department of Life and Health Sciences, University of Nicosia, Nicosia, Cyprus

Shamma Ebrahim AlZaabi
Health and Safety Department, UAE Armed Forces, GHQ, Abu Dhabi, United Arab Emirates

Munawwar Ali Khan
Department of Life and Environmental Sciences, College of Natural and Health Sciences, Zayed University, Dubai, United Arab Emirates

Ludmilla F. Wikkeling-Scott
Assistant Professor, Zayed University, College of Natural and Health Sciences, Department of Health Sciences

R.V. Rikard
Senior Postdoctoral Research Associate, Michigan State University, Department of Media and Information

Sirine Maher Zahran
Department of Natural Sciences and Public Health, Zayed University, Abu Dhabi, UAE

Zainab Taha
College of Natural and Health Sciences, Zayed University, Abu Dhabi, U.A.E.

Nada Salhab
Maastricht University, Minderbroedersberg 4-6, 6211 LK Maastricht, The Netherlands

Mirey Karavetian
Zayed University, Academic City - Dubai, United Arab Emirates

Jeroen Kooman
University Hospital Maastricht, P. Debyelaan 25, 6229 HX Maastricht, The Netherlands

Enrico Fiaccadori
Parma University, Via Università, 12, 43121 Parma PR, Italy

Lalia Chrara, Riad A. Raoui, Adel Belkadi and Othman Benbernou
Laboratory for Optimising Research Programmes on Physical and Sports Activities, University of Mostaganem, Algeria

Hocine Asli
Institute of Physical Education and Sport, University of Oran, Mostaganem, Algeria

Marcou Juliana and Savva Rafaella-Maria
Department of Life and Health Sciences, University of Nicosia, Nicosia, Cyprus

Michalis Anastasiadis
Department of Life & Health Sciences, University of Nicosia, 46, Makedonitissas Avenue, Nicosia, Cyprus

Thomas Kourtessis
Department of Physical Education & Sport Science, Democritus University of Thrace, University Campus, Komotini, Greece

Evridiki Zachopoulou
Department of Early Childhood Care and Education, Alexander Technological Educational Institute of Thessaloniki, Greece

Sousana Papadopoulou, Elpiniki Kroustalloudi, Anna Kokkinopoulou and Maria Hassapidou
Department of Nutrition & Dietetics, Alexander Technological Educational Institute of Thessaloniki, Sindos, Thessaloniki, Greece

Shaima K. AlBlooshi and Lina T. Al Kury
Deartment of Health Sciences, Zayed University, Abu Dhabi, United Arab Emirates

Pavlos Malindretos
General Hospital of Volos, Volos, Greece

Index

www.ingramcontent.com/pod-product-compliance
Lightning Source LLC
LaVergne TN
LVHW060526210926
848485LV00005B/1153
* 9 7 8 1 6 3 9 8 9 0 4 5 3 *